**TAKE CHARGE OF YOUR ASTHMA AND
ENJOY YOUR LIFE. GET THE ANSWERS TO
THESE AND OTHER IMPORTANT QUESTIONS:**

—What are the warning signs of an oncoming attack?
—How can a woman with asthma have a successful
  pregnancy?
—Do allergies trigger asthma attacks?
—What if a person with asthma needs surgery?
—Can people with asthma have pets?
—Are there ways to tell if foods can cause asthma at-
  tacks?

Living with Asthma

Anthony Rooklin, M.D., has written extensively
about pulmonary disorders, allergies, and immunology. He received his medical degree from Thomas
Jefferson University School of Medicine in 1972.
Shelagh Ryan Masline is an experienced writer and
editor in the field of health.

LIVING

WITH

Asthma

*A Comprehensive Guide to
Understanding and Controlling Asthma
While Enjoying Your Life*

ANTHONY R. ROOKLIN, M.D.
AND
SHELAGH RYAN MASLINE

Illustrations by Kent Humphreys

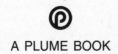

A PLUME BOOK

A NOTE TO THE READER

The ideas, procedures, and suggestions contained in this book are not intended as a substitute for consulting with your physician. All matters regarding your health require medical supervision.

PLUME
Published by the Penguin Group
Penguin Books USA Inc., 375 Hudson Street,
New York, New York 10014, U.S.A.
Penguin Books Ltd, 27 Wrights Lane, London W8 5TZ, England
Penguin Books Australia Ltd, Ringwood, Victoria, Australia
Penguin Books Canada Ltd, 10 Alcorn Avenue,
Toronto, Ontario, Canada M4V 3B2
Penguin Books (N.Z.) Ltd, 182–190 Wairau Road,
Auckland 10, New Zealand

Penguin Books Ltd, Registered Offices:
Harmondsworth, Middlesex, England

First published by Plume, an imprint of Dutton Signet,
a division of Penguin Books USA Inc.

First Printing, January, 1995
10 9 8 7 6 5 4 3 2

 REGISTERED TRADEMARK—MARCA REGISTRADA

LIBRARY OF CONGRESS CATALOGING-IN-PUBLICATION DATA:
Rooklin, Anthony R.
    Living with asthma / Anthony R. Rooklin and Shelagh Ryan Masline;
illustrations by Kent Humphreys.
    p. cm.
    ISBN 0-452-27250-5
    1. Asthma—Popular works. I. Masline, Shelagh A. R.   II. Title.
RC591.R66 1995
616.2'38—dc20   94–18487
                                                                    CIP

Printed in the United States of America
Set in Century Expanded
Designed by Eve L. Kirch

Contents

Foreword

Many of the patients who come to me for treatment are asthmatics. It is my goal to change them into normal people who happen to have asthma. My definition of a normal person is someone who sleeps through the night, wakes up with a clear chest in the morning, attends school or work daily, and can enjoy all the exercise he or she wants.

Asthma is an extremely treatable disease that should not infringe excessively upon your life. I see myself as one who can help patients learn what they need to do to lead as normal a life as anyone else despite the fact that they have asthma.

Asthma has many faces. Wheezing, coughing, tightness in the chest, and congestion may all be signs that you have asthma. Many people suffer from the symptoms of asthma and don't even know it. Maybe you have a nagging cough or a tendency to develop bronchitis whenever you get a cold—and maybe you have asthma.

Aggressive treatment with asthma medications, which are increasingly effective and relatively free of side effects, can help. But the right diagnosis has to be made before treatment can begin.

I never discourage my patients from engaging in the sport or exercise of their choice. Running, playing basketball or soccer, doing aerobics: except in very rare cases, you can do them all, provided you have the proper medication. You can also enjoy a normal pregnancy or undergo surgery despite your asthma—as long as your asthma is well controlled.

To help my patients understand their disease, I often compare asthma to the glowing embers in a barbecue pit. Imagine these embers as the inflammation in the airways inside your lungs. The embers flare up when fuel is poured on them—that is, when the symptoms of your asthma are triggered by such things as allergies, upper-respiratory infections, exercise, cigarette smoke, or changes in the weather. You can put out the flare-up of asthma symptoms by using a bronchodilator, which is like a fire extinguisher. Even more effectively, doctors can treat the underlying inflammation of asthma and prevent symptoms from occurring: anti-inflammatory medications, when used regularly, can cool down the glowing embers of hyperreactive airways.

Many patients with asthma think it's normal to wheeze, have a persistent cough, or wake up during the night to use a bronchodilator. In this book you will learn that this is *not* normal. When your asthma is well controlled, you do not have to tolerate these symptoms.

This book is about how *well* you can be with asthma. Doctors can and must educate their patients to understand their asthma and manage their condition as effectively as possible. If you use your bronchodilating inhaler more than four times a day, you are probably tolerating more symptoms than you should. In these and other cases, which we will tell you about in this book, it may be necessary to reach beyond your primary-care physician and see an asthma specialist. Most importantly, we want you to learn how to recognize and control the symptoms of your asthma. When your asthma is well controlled, you are more likely to enjoy a full and normal life.

—ANTHONY R. ROOKLIN, M.D.

CHAPTER 1

Fact vs. Fiction

Is it suddenly harder to catch your breath after you run up a flight of stairs? Do you find yourself struggling for a gulp of fresh air after a workout or jog? Maybe you're a bit worried about that wheezing, whistling sound that accompanies your breathing—or the alarming tightness in your chest when the family cat strolls through the room.

What about your children? Does your toddler's breathing seem unusually labored whenever she gets a cold? Does your five-year-old seem to tire more quickly than his friends? Is he unusually sensitive to cold air, or does he have a difficult time breathing during pollen season?

Many of us put off a visit to the doctor, hoping that we can simply ignore discomforts like these and they will go away. Others of us feel we can live with a nagging cough, or put up with being short of breath. We don't like to think of ourselves as less than well. But if you (or your child) experience problems such as the ones we've just mentioned, you may be among the 12 million Americans who have the very treatable disease known as asthma.

There is no reason for you to suffer from the symptoms of asthma. You don't have to "put up" with anything! The medicines we use to relieve asthma symptoms are safe, effective, and getting better all the time. You and your doctor can team up to identify what triggers your asthma, and you can work together to come up with strategies to avoid or, when necessary, cope with these triggers. If an allergic response to dust or pollen sets off your asthmatic episodes, you may be able to avoid them; if you're a runner and exercise brings on your asthma, your doctor can provide the medication your body requires to run without discomfort. After all, asthma hasn't slowed down Olympic runner Jackie Joyner-Kersee.

Except in rare cases, asthma should not prevent you from pursuing any reasonable activity you want to. When in doubt, asthma specialists are available to complement the treatment of your regular doctor in providing state-of-the-art care. Understanding your asthma is the first step toward managing your disease and enjoying a better quality of life. Let's start out by clearing up some common misconceptions about asthma.

MYTH: Asthma is just in your head.
FACT: Let's debunk this old folk tale right away. Asthma is not a psychosomatic disease. It is a chronic and potentially very serious lung condition.

MYTH: Asthma is caused by stress.
FACT: Stress does not *cause* asthma—but asthma can lead to anxiety or emotional problems, especially in those who have not learned how to cope with their con-

dition. Strong emotions may also trigger asthma symptoms, but they can't do so unless you already have asthma. Asthma is in your lungs—not in your head.

MYTH: Allergies are the same as asthma.

FACT: Allergies can bring on asthma symptoms, and the relationship between allergies and asthma is very close. But not *all* asthmatics have allergies, and not everyone who has allergies has asthma. While an asthmatic person has a very specific lung problem, an allergic individual is someone whose immune system has become sensitized to normally harmless substances called allergens.

MYTH: People with asthma need to live restricted lives.

FACT: Many people just tolerate their symptoms. They think it is normal to wheeze, have a persistent cough, or wake up during the middle of the night to relieve their asthma symptoms with a bronchodilator. This is not normal! Give yourself a break and find out just how well you can be with the appropriate treatment. People with asthma should be able to sleep through the night and awaken with a clear chest in the morning. They should not have to miss school or work or restrict their activity.

MYTH: People with asthma should not exercise.

FACT: If you have asthma, you *should* exercise. Exercise can actually help your asthma by improving your aerobic conditioning. This misconception probably arises because exercise is a common *trigger* of asthma symptoms. If exercise is a trigger for *your* asthma, work with your doctor to learn how to pace yourself. Your doctor may also prescribe medications you can take before exercising to prevent symptoms.

MYTH: Asthma is a disease of young people.
FACT: Asthma is a disease of all ages. Although it is true that asthma is most common in children, it can occur at any time of life. In fact, when people over the age of sixty get asthma, they are often undertreated or inappropriately diagnosed as having emphysema or bronchitis.

MYTH: Children outgrow asthma.
FACT: It is true that the symptoms of asthma may diminish and even disappear as children grow older. But it's important to keep in mind that once you have the hyperreactive, or "twitchy," airways of asthma, under certain conditions—such as when you move into a new apartment or get a pet—these symptoms can recur.

MYTH: Asthma is the same as emphysema.
FACT: Elderly people who have asthma are sometimes misdiagnosed as having emphysema. But although the shortness of breath and wheezing of emphysema may mimic the symptoms of asthma, these are actually two very different diseases. Emphysema, which usually follows a lifetime of cigarette smoking, is a progressive disease that permanently damages the air sacs of the lungs. Asthma is a *reversible* disease of the bronchioles, which open into the air sacs. (We'll explain this in more detail in Chapter 2.)

MYTH: Asthma is a fatal disease.
FACT: No asthma attack need be fatal. Asthma is a very treatable disease. On the other hand, asthma must

be taken very seriously, because *without* proper treatment it can be fatal. The most up-to-date approach to asthma is self-management. Even very young patients are encouraged to take an active role in their continuing care—and with the aggressive forms of treatment available today, it's increasingly clear that asthma sufferers can live long, full lives.

CHAPTER 2

What Is Asthma?

When you can't breathe—when you're wheezing and coughing and you can't figure out why—it's time to visit your doctor and find out whether you have asthma. Asthma is a disease of the lungs involving reversible blockage of the airways and chronic inflammation. The most common symptoms caused by this blockage and inflammation are wheezing, coughing, chest tightness, and shortness of breath. But the good news is that asthma is reversible: medication can prevent and, when necessary, relieve these and other symptoms.

Asthma is one of the most common chronic illnesses, yet it is also one of the most frequently undertreated. Unfortunately—and sometimes tragically—while scientific advances are making it easier than ever to live with asthma, the message doesn't seem to be getting out to everyone:

- Experts believe that some 12 million Americans suffer from asthma. More than $1 billion is spent each year on health care for asthma, according to the American College of Allergy and Immunology in Arlington Heights, Illinois. In fact, estimates made by the National Institutes of Health put health care costs for asthma at more than $4 billion in 1988.

• The National Jewish Center for Immunology and Respiratory Medicine, a world leader in the treatment of asthma, points out that chronic respiratory disease is the leading cause of absenteeism from school and work and the most frequent reason people seek medical care.

• Asthma cases increased by 29 percent between 1980 and 1987, according to the National Institutes of Health. Even more alarming, death rates from asthma increased by 31 percent during that time.

When you look at these statistics, it becomes increasingly clear that learning how to understand and manage your asthma may be the most valuable lesson of your life. Although there is no cure for asthma, many effective treatments are available to control and reverse this chronic disease. Let's take a look at who gets asthma, what happens inside your lungs when you have the disease, and how you can get it under control.

Who Gets Asthma?

People of any age, ethnic group, race, or cultural background can have asthma. Although no one knows exactly what causes it, we do know that people with asthma have certain things in common. Most importantly, asthma has a genetic basis: it tends to occur in families. A child whose parents have asthma is far more likely to develop the disease than the child of nonasthmatic parents.

Although you can get asthma at any age, it is most likely to turn up for the first time in children under the age of five. More than half of all asthma cases are found in children between the ages of two and seventeen. Until puberty, boys are almost twice as likely to get asthma as girls, although no one knows exactly why. Another aspect of asthma is that it is especially common in African-Americans.

To develop asthma, experts believe that you must be born with some genetic predisposition to the disease. Everyone with asthma has some degree of inflammation in the airways, as well as hyperreactive, or "twitchy," airways that can go into bronchospasm when exposed to triggers. But not everyone with a predisposition to asthma develops the condition. Asthma symptoms are triggered by various factors, such as allergens, irritants, infections, pollutants, medications, and emotions.

The Triggers of Asthma

Triggers are substances or situations that would be quite harmless to people with ordinary airways, but that bring on asthma symptoms in susceptible individuals. Triggers vary widely from person to person. There is a very close correlation, for example, between asthma and allergies. In young children, common triggers of asthma are colds and other upper-respiratory infections.

Allergens, viral respiratory infections, aspirin, occupational hazards, physical exertion, food additives, and irritants such as cigarette smoke—any of these, alone or in combination, may trigger asthma symptoms.

Learning the triggers of asthma is a key part of understanding the disease, and we will study them in detail in the next chapter.

Asthma Is Reversible

Asthma cases are widely variable: a mild case may manifest itself as an annoying cough, but a severe asthma attack can send you off to the hospital emergency room to relieve an acute blockage of your airways. But the most critical feature that almost all cases of asthma have in common is their *reversibility*. Quite literally, this means that doctors can reverse the symptoms of asthma. We can handle this disease; you can control your asthma.

Specialists emphasize that it is important to think positively: don't be frightened of your asthma. It is true that, left untreated, asthma can be a dangerous and indeed life-threatening condition, but doctors today have medications to reverse and even prevent the blockage of your airways, enabling you to breathe freely once more.

The worst thing you can do is ignore your asthma. Don't overlook or put up with the discomfort—and the possible long-term consequences for your health—of wheezing, coughing, and shortness of breath. The best thing you can do is to consult your regular doctor or asthma specialists and obtain the excellent care that is available today. You will find that the more you learn about your asthma, the less frightened and better equipped you will be to manage it. To help you understand just what is happening in your lungs when the symptoms of asthma occur, let's take a look at how the normal breathing process works.

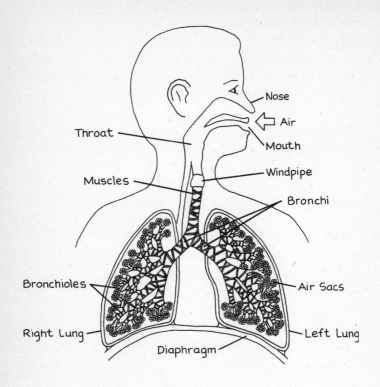

Illustration 1. The Respiratory System

The Normal Breathing Process

Take a deep breath. Breathe in, breathe out. It sounds so simple, and it is for most people. In the normal breathing process the lungs accomplish an essential exchange: they take in the oxygen from the air to nourish the body and dispose of the waste product carbon dioxide. This is the vital function we call respiration.

"Respiration" comes from the Latin *respirare*, which means "to respire or breathe."

Fresh air first enters through the nose, which acts as a kind of filter and humidifier. A sticky coating of mucus traps and removes dust, germs, and other impurities. This filtering system is one of the body's natural ways of protecting itself, by cleaning air as fully as possible before it enters the lungs.

Air then passes down through the windpipe, or trachea, into the lungs. Now, picture a series of branches in each of your lungs, which you can think of as upside-down trees. The trachea first divides into two large air tubes called bronchi, and the bronchus ("bronchus" is the singular of "bronchi") forms the trunk of the upside-down tree in each lung. The bronchi continue to branch out through the lungs, growing progressively smaller, until they reach the smallest bronchi, which are known as bronchioles.

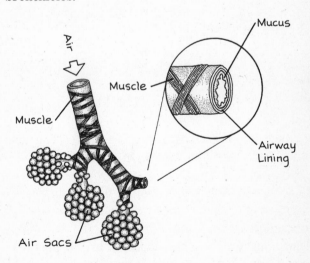

Illustration 2. A Normal Bronchial Tube

The smallest bronchioles eventually open into tiny balloon-like air sacs called alveoli. A thin membrane separates the alveoli from the blood vessels of the lung, and it is here that the essential exchange of oxygen and carbon dioxide takes place. Indispensable oxygen from fresh air is absorbed through the membrane into small blood vessels called capillaries, while the waste product carbon dioxide passes from the blood to the alveoli, and on out through the bronchioles, bronchi, trachea, and nose. All these things happen as you breathe out in a normal exhalation.

Each component of the lungs plays a key role in respiration. But the parts of the lungs we're most concerned with here are those that asthma affects: the airways, or bronchi and bronchioles, which are the breathing tubes inside the lungs. Take another deep breath. Breathe in, breathe out. When you have asthma, sometimes this is not so easy after all. To help you understand why, we'll explore what happens inside an asthmatic lung.

The Asthmatic Lung

Difficulty in breathing, shortness of breath, coughing, congestion, wheezing, tightness in the chest—if you have asthma, you may encounter any one or a combination of these symptoms. Some people have chronic symptoms every day: others experience seasonal symptoms or occasional acute episodes.

The underlying basis of asthma in the lungs is the same in any case, varying mainly in severity. When asthma symptoms are triggered, we know that three major events are taking place inside the lungs to block the flow of air through them:

- An inflammatory response recruits a variety of cells into the bronchial tubes, which can lead to blockage of the bronchi and thickening of the inside walls of the bronchial tubes.
- The smooth muscles that surround the bronchi are hyperreactive, or "twitchy." When triggered, the muscles tighten, narrowing the air passages and reducing the flow of air through them.
- Glands inside the airways clog already narrowed air passages by excreting excessive amounts of thick and sticky mucus.

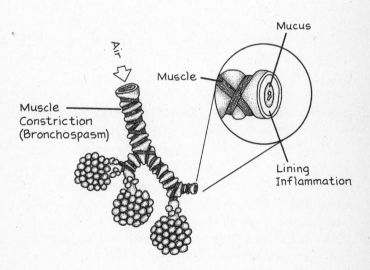

Illustration 3. A Bronchial Tube During an Asthmatic Episode

Asthma: An Inflammatory Disease

As recently as ten years ago, doctors tended to concentrate mainly on "asthma attacks," acute episodes of airway blockage. But recent studies have found that the most universal and potentially most dangerous aspect of asthma is the inflammation taking place in the airways.

One of the most important things you can do is to work with your doctor to manage the inflammation of asthma. We've pointed out that asthma is reversible—but you must take measures to reverse it, primarily by limiting your exposure to substances that trigger your symptoms and by taking appropriate medication.

Inflammation of the airway linings is triggered by various stimuli, such as allergens (house-dust mites, molds, animal dander, etc.) or environmental irritants (cigarette smoke, certain perfumes, cleaning products, etc.). Cells lining the airways respond to the trigger by releasing chemical substances known as mediators, which lead to inflammation. The airway linings swell, the smooth muscles contract, and the airways are narrowed.

Specialists today recommend that most people with asthma take anti-inflammatory drugs such as cromolyn sodium or inhaled steroids regularly, even when symptoms are not present. (We'll discuss these drugs in Chapter 8.) Experts judge that too much emphasis has been placed on relieving symptoms, while not enough attention has been paid to preventing them.

Anti-inflammatory drugs are now used in a way similar to drugs prescribed to control hypertension, or high blood pressure. Like high blood pressure, inflammation inside the airways can do its silent damage slowly, over a long period. The longer you allow inflammation to remain out of control, the more lung damage you risk. Using preventive drugs routinely can control underlying inflammation. Furthermore, medical studies show that treatment of airway inflammation reduces the hyperreactivity of the airways and prevents asthma attacks.

Asthma: A Reactive Airway Disease

When you have asthma, you have what doctors refer to as hyperreactive, or twitchy, airways. Asthmatic airways are extremely sensitive to a wide variety of triggers, such as allergens, environmental irritants, upper-respiratory infections, exercise, and cold air. Triggers differ from person to person: pollen might set off symptoms in Jane, while animal hair is the real problem for John. But whatever your triggers may be, your bronchioles become irritated when exposed to them.

Airways are surrounded by bands of smooth muscles, which look much like the stripes on a candy cane. The asthmatic lung responds to ordinary substances—such as the pollen or animal hair mentioned above—as hostile invaders, and it takes action to rid the body of them. When triggers enter the lungs, muscles tighten around the airways in an attempt to expel them. This results in a muscle spasm around the airways, called a bronchospasm.

Muscle constriction joins inflammation to further narrow the airways and block the flow of air. The consequent symptoms may be mild, severe, or anywhere in between. For example, a mild case of asthma might manifest itself as occasional shortness of breath during pollen seasons. On the other hand, in severe cases of asthma, as less and less air is able to enter your lungs, you may experience an asthma attack. After we explore the third component of asthma, we'll take a closer look at asthma attacks.

Asthma: A Condition of Clogged Airways

The third component of asthma is the excessive output of mucus in the airways. The mucus membrane extends from the nose, mouth, and trachea into the airways of the lungs. Normally this mucus lining is very useful to the body. As we mentioned earlier, before air reaches the lungs mucus acts to remove impurities from it.

But when you have asthma, mucus can become a problem. In many cases of asthma, as part of the inflammatory response excessive amounts of thick mucus are secreted from the cells of the mucus membrane, clogging the airways and making it even harder to breathe.

That old cold remedy—drinking plenty of fluids—is one way of naturally coping with excess mucus production. Unfortunately, this doesn't do the trick for everyone. Your doctors may prescribe expectorants, which thin mucus and make it easier for you to cough it up. In other instances, corticosteroid medications are recommended to decrease the inflammation that can lead to this elevation in mucus production. (Again, these drugs will be discussed in Chapter 8.)

What Is an Asthma Attack?

Asthma attacks are the feature of asthma you've probably heard most about, and many people have an understandable fear of these episodes. But asthma attacks, like less serious symptoms of asthma, can be prevented in many cases—and when they do occur, they can be controlled.

In an asthma attack, you become progressively short of breath, and may find yourself gulping, gasping, and wheezing as you try to fill the cramped airways of your lungs with air. You may feel as if you're suffocating. Signs of panic, such as sweating, dizziness, and rapid heartbeat, often accompany asthma attacks.

An Airway Obstruction

An asthma attack, which may last moments or days, is the result of a severe airway obstruction, which is in turn caused by some combination of the three components of asthma. Symptoms seem to develop suddenly in an asthma attack. Inflammation inside the airways of the lungs is joined by the contraction of muscles around the airways, which reduces the flow of air through them. Airways may narrow even further because of excess mucus production. The most severe and prolonged asthma attack is known as status asthmaticus, a condition that requires hospitalization for special treatment.

Warning Signs

An asthma attack can be very frightening—especially the first one—but you can learn to recognize the warning signs of an attack. The signals differ from person to person. Besides the increased coughing and wheezing that accompany difficulty in breathing, you may experience tiredness, headache, moodiness, sneezing, or itching in the throat area.

Preventing an Asthma Attack

Once you learn to recognize the warning signs of your asthma attacks, you can take precautions to head off an attack or at least lessen its severity. Your doctor will work with you to determine your best strategy. As in all cases of asthma, your best bet is usually a combination of avoiding exposure to triggers and taking anti-inflammatory drugs as preventive medication.

Relieving an Asthma Attack

Sometimes, despite all the precautions you take, you have an asthma attack. Fortunately, medications known as bronchodilators can relieve an attack. These medications can be taken as liquids, as pills, or by inhalation. Today most bronchodilator medications are taken using metered-dose inhalers, also known as MDIs or puffers. These are small hand-held devices through which you breath in the medication. Bronchodilators ease the acute symptoms of an asthma attack by opening the airways, relaxing the smooth muscles, and decreasing the sensitivity of the airways. (We'll discuss the proper use of inhalers, as well as the pros and cons of different bronchodilator medications, in Chapter 8.)

Emergency Treatment of an Asthma Attack

If bronchodilator medication is not on hand to treat a severe asthma attack, your skin may begin to look bluish as your oxygen supply is cut off. Don't waste time: go straight to your doctor's office or to the emergency room. If you have a car, drive there, or better yet have someone else drive you. If you don't have a car, dial 911.

The most common emergency treatments for an asthma attack are an injection of epinephrine (Adrenalin) or a breathing treatment using similar medicine, both of which usually produce a dramatic improvement in breathing almost instantly. It is most important that you discuss with your doctor beforehand how and when to use bronchodilator medication. Having a well-thought-out emergency plan will allow you to avoid the anxiety that often accompanies the patient with a diagnosis of asthma. Knowing when to contact your physician—so that you can increase your medication early in the attack—will almost always help you control your asthma flare-up and prevent a visit to the emergency room. (Turn to Chapter 8 for more information on the treatment of asthma attacks.)

Controlling Your Asthma

It's important to remember—whether you are young or old and whether your asthma is mild or severe—that doctors today have the knowledge and tools to work with you to control your asthma. In June 1991 the National Institutes of Health published a new set of guidelines for the diagnosis and management of asthma, emphasizing closer monitoring of lung function and greater attention to the airway inflammation that underlies all cases of asthma. The report describes four major ways in which you and your doctor can work together to diagnose your asthma and keep it under control. These four steps can help virtually everyone with asthma lead a normal and productive life.

- The first step is getting an accurate diagnosis of your asthma. Besides taking a detailed medical history, your doctor will use objective measures of lung function to both diagnose and monitor your asthma. (In Chapter 4 we'll describe these breathing tests, which measure the level of obstruction in the airways.) Objective measures are especially important in asthma management, because often your symptoms—and sometimes even your doctor's physical examination—do not tell the whole story.

- Once you know you have asthma, your doctor will prescribe appropriate medication for you to use regularly. Asthma medications are safe and effective, and your doctor will determine the medications that best suit your case. It's important to remember how and when to take all medications, and not to skip doses. (For a complete discussion of the medications used to treat asthma, turn to Chapter 8.)

- It is vital to work with your doctor to identify and avoid the triggers that bring on your asthma symptoms. As we have said, there are many different triggers—such as allergies and upper-respiratory infections—and they vary from person to person. Avoiding and, when possible, eliminating these triggers from your life is a key part of asthma management. (Read more about these triggers in Chapter 3.)

• You must build a partnership with your doctor, family, and close friends to help control your asthma. Experts recognize that much of the everyday burden of asthma management falls on your shoulders, and it's a big job. The understanding and support of those around you can be a great help in developing the motivation and practical skills to stay on top of your asthma.

Asthma and Other Lung Problems

Repeated bouts of coughing and wheezing are most likely caused by asthma, but there are a number of asthma lookalikes—other lung conditions that resemble asthma—and these must be ruled out as the cause of your symptoms before your doctor conclusively determines that asthma is the problem. A number of visits to your doctor may be necessary to confirm the diagnosis. Following are a few lung problems that are commonly mistaken for asthma.

An Obstruction of the Airways

If a foreign object becomes lodged in one of your lungs, the consequent lung inflammation and wheezing can make it look as though you have asthma. An astonishing array of objects has been removed from people's lungs—ranging from peanuts to peach pits to cigarette butts to hairballs! Although adults and older children are usually aware of having a foreign body in the lung, infants and young children may aspirate something unknown to anyone else.

A key to diagnosing this kind of airway obstruction is that the problem will show up only in one lung. Asthma, on the other hand, affects both your lungs. A chest X ray can help pinpoint the problem. A careful and thorough medical history and a high index of suspicion will usually allow the physician to make the correct diagnosis.

Cardiac Asthma

Older people who seem to have asthma may actually suffer from a condition called cardiac asthma, which is not asthma at all. In this case, asthma-like symptoms, such as wheezing, are caused by heart failure. The wheezing is caused by a buildup of fluid in the lungs, and is brought on by the heart's failure to pump blood efficiently.

Heart failure may be suspected if the patient is elderly and has not previously suffered from asthma. Besides wheezing in the lungs, the symptoms brought on by heart failure include swollen ankles and bulging veins in the neck. A chest X ray, the key to diagnosis, will reveal the fluid in the lungs and enlarged heart typical of heart failure. It is important to remember that increasing respiratory difficulty in a patient with asthma may be caused by something other than asthma.

Chronic Bronchitis

Chronic bronchitis, which is characterized by a persistent mucus-producing cough, is most often found in people who smoke or who live or work in polluted areas. The mucus can become infected, requiring treatment with antibiotics. Bronchodilators may help such people breathe, although some of the damage may be irreversible. Diagnosis is usually made through taking a careful medical history, including a smoking history, breathing tests, and chest X ray.

Cystic Fibrosis

Cystic fibrosis is an extremely serious childhood disease that is sometimes mistaken for asthma. Children with cystic fibrosis experience recurrent lung infections, which are associated with excessive mucus production and may eventually cause serious lung damage. Since cystic fibrosis can be present with symptoms similar to those of asthma, diagnosis may be difficult. A sweat chloride test will determine whether a child is suffering from cystic fibrosis.

Emphysema

Emphysema is a very serious disease that usually affects middle-aged and older individuals and causes permanent damage to the walls of the air sacs inside the lungs. Like chronic bronchitis, it is usually associated with long years of cigarette smoking or constant exposure to pollution in the air. Emphysema is characterized by shortness of breath and a persistent, dry cough.

Unlike asthma, emphysema is not reversible. It is a severely disabling disease, in which shortness of breath gets progressively worse. Chest X rays and breathing tests can determine whether a person suffers from emphysema. Treatment requires an immediate cessation of smoking, and when the emphysema is severe often involves regular inhalation of supplementary oxygen. Asthma and emphysema may coexist in the same patient. Although the emphysema may be untreatable, when the asthma component is aggressively treated, the patient will often feel much better and experience an improved quality of life.

CHAPTER 3

The Triggers
of Asthma

Triggers are ordinary substances or events that have no special impact on people who do not have asthma. But airways in the lungs of asthmatics are subject to chronic inflammation. This inflammation makes the airways unusually sensitive to environmental stimulants, which can set off one or more of the symptoms of asthma: shortness of breath, wheezing, coughing, and tightness in the chest.

The triggers of asthma vary from person to person. A trigger that brings on shortness of breath in one asthmatic may have no affect at all on another. There are also many different triggers of asthma, such as allergies, airborne irritants, viral respiratory tract infections (colds and flu), reactions to certain forms of exercise, strong emotions, and aspirin sensitivity.

Identifying and coping with the triggers of asthma, along with taking appropriate medication, is the key to successful asthma management. But the first step is to work with your doctor to identify the triggers of your particular case. Following are descriptions of some of the more common triggers of asthma. (Turn to Chapter 7 for practical advice on how to avoid or control asthma triggers.)

Allergies

The close connection between allergies and asthma has long been recognized, but it's important to remember that allergies and asthma are two different conditions. Asthma, as we've explained, is a reversible obstruction of the airways or bronchial tubes inside the lungs. Allergies, a common trigger of asthma symptoms, occur when the immune system becomes sensitized to ordinarily harmless substances known as allergens. Specialists pay careful attention to allergies as they diagnose and treat asthma.

Allergens most commonly bring reactions involving the skin, blood vessels, digestive system, and respiratory system. The allergens that normally affect people with asthma are those that are inhaled. Foods, for example, are occasional but not frequent triggers of asthma. Substances that enter the air we breathe—outdoor allergens, such as grass and ragweed pollen, and indoor allergens, such as dust mites and cockroach droppings—are the usual culprits. And whether indoors or out, mold spores, animal dander, and feathers are inhaled substances that can bring on allergic reactions.

A Genetic Predisposition

People who are allergy-prone, or atopic, have a genetic predisposition to manufacture large amounts of antibodies known as immunoglobulin E (IgE). Being atopic is closely linked to both allergies and asthma. It is the exposure of atopic individuals to allergens that stimulates the production of IgE; when the allergen and specific IgE for the allergen link together, certain cells called mast cells are directed to discharge substances that can bring on the symptoms of asthma.

Although the tendencies to manufacture IgE and experience allergic reactions are hereditary, or genetic, *specific* allergies are not actually passed on. Your mother, for example, might have eczema (a skin problem), while allergies manifest themselves in you as hay fever (a respiratory problem).

An Allergic Reaction

An allergy is an overreaction of your immune system to a substance that is harmless to other people. The immune system generally offers protection from dangerous materials, but when you have allergies, your immune system "protects" you from normally benign substances.

We all have white blood cells called mast cells in the nose, air passages, and skin. Mast cells play a major role in the development of allergies in atopic individuals. The initial phase of an allergic reaction happens when mast cells are exposed and sensitized to a particular allergen, such as dust mites, animal dander, pollen, or mold spores. This first exposure of the mast cells does not cause an allergic reaction, but *repeated* exposure or sensitization to the allergen causes allergies to develop.

When your immune system perceives a substance entering your body as a hostile invader, it stimulates white blood cells to respond to the invader in an effort to protect your body. The white blood cells we mentioned above, mast cells, are coated with IgE antibodies specific to a variety of allergens. When an IgE antibody in the mast cells' surface comes into contact with an allergen, the mast cells release protective chemicals known as mediators.

Mediators bring on allergic symptoms—such as sneezing, a runny nose, or a sinus headache—and can also trigger asthma symptoms in susceptible individuals. One of the mediators specific to asthma is histamine. The mediators not only cause immediate symptoms, they also stimulate an influx of certain inflammatory white cells that can cause symptoms several hours after the exposure. The inflammation caused by these cells can make the airways hyperreactive, or twitchy. The more severe the inflammation, the more severe the immediate reaction when you are exposed to allergens.

House-Dust Mites

Dust mites are common allergens that often induce the symptoms of allergies and asthma. The house-dust mite is a lilliputian bug that feeds off skin cells and tiny specks of food. You'd have to look under a microscope to see these insects, but the havoc they can wreak in your body is all out of proportion to their size.

Children who grow up in houses where there are many dust mites are far more likely to develop asthma than children from homes free of dust mites. Cleanliness should be a priority of families who have a history of allergies or asthma, and it's a good idea to remove from the home dust-collectors such as heavy carpeting or drapes. (Practical tips on keeping your home allergy- and asthma-proof are included in Chapter 7.)

Animal Dander, Bird Droppings, and Feathers

Pets can be our companions and provide love, comfort, and security. On the other hand, having a pet is often difficult for people who suffer from allergies or asthma. Pets may cause allergic problems that lead to asthma, and they can do so both directly and indirectly. Animal dander, or flakes of skin, can cause an allergic reaction in susceptible people, as can the saliva or urine of a pet. The hair and fur of animals may also indirectly cause symptoms, as they collect dust, pollen, and other allergens.

Seasonal Allergies

Tree and grass pollen and mold spores plague allergy sufferers each spring; ragweed joins mold spores to cause symptoms in many people in the fall. Patterns vary, of course, from region to region, and if you experience seasonal symptoms you should ask your doctor to confirm the seasonal pattern where you live.

Although seasonal allergies may prompt you to consider a move, it's important to keep in mind that your genetic predisposition toward allergies does not disappear when you make a geographical relocation. Moving is a drastic and often ineffective answer. If your asthma is brought on by allergies, you may find that it is only a matter of time before you are exposed to different allergens in your new home, and in response develop new allergies that can trigger asthma symptoms.

Do Allergies Play a Role in Your Asthma?

To determine whether allergies are a trigger for your asthma, ask yourself the following questions. One or more "yes" answers indicates that allergies may play a role in your asthma.

- Is your asthma worse in certain months?
- Do asthma symptoms occur when you visit friends who have pets?
- If you have a pet, do symptoms improve when you spend time away from home?
- Does your asthma get worse when dust is raised as you vacuum?
- Do you develop asthma symptoms when you visit a barn or stable?
- Do you experience asthma symptoms in damp basements or poorly ventilated bathrooms?
- Are your asthma symptoms brought on by your work environment or by performing certain tasks at your job?

Testing for Allergies

Allergies are often determined by your doctor through a detailed medical history. But if there is any doubt, the next step is usually skin testing for allergens by a board-certified allergist. This will settle whether or not you have allergies and, if you do, which allergens are the ones that affect you.

The allergist conducts a skin test by pricking your arm or back with a needle and applying a diluted allergen solution. The pinprick is tiny and not very painful. If you do have an allergy to that substance, the skin around the pinprick will redden and a small hive or welt will form within minutes. This means that the IgE antibodies specific to the allergen have responded by triggering a release of histamine and other mediators from the mast cells.

A skin test is the most common way in which doctors determine allergies. An alternative to skin testing is a blood test known as RAST (Radioallergosorbent Test). This test, which is more expensive and time-consuming than skin tests, measures allergen-specific IgE antibodies in the blood.

Exercise

Exercise is one of the best things you can do for your asthma: exercise boosts respiratory capacity and adds to an overall sense of well-being. But exercise must be monitored by your doctor, since unregulated exercise often leads to wheezing and coughing.

Many people begin to breathe more rapidly through their mouths while exercising. The air that reaches the bronchial tubes inside the lungs through the mouth is not as warmed and humidified as the air that passes through the nose. Cold, dry air, in combination with the larger amounts of air taken in while exercising, may irritate twitchy airways and trigger asthma symptoms. Fortunately, preventive treatment can help most asthmatics enjoy the exercise of their choice. (Read more about asthma and exercise in Chapter 9.)

Upper-Respiratory Infections

Upper-respiratory viral infections, such as the flu and the common cold, are another major trigger of asthma symptoms, especially in children. A tight chest, shortness of breath, and wheezing often follow the congestion of colds and sore throats in children. Infections cause irritation and increase bronchial sensitivity. Since viruses are the most frequent cause of upper-respiratory infections, antibiotics do not help. (Antibiotics can cure only bacterial infections—not viruses.) Try to take preventive measures, such as getting flu shots and frequently washing your own and your child's hands to avoid passing on viruses.

Nocturnal Asthma

Worsening of asthma at night, or nocturnal asthma, is very frequent in asthmatics. There are a number of possible reasons for this:

- Medication may wear off late at night or early in the morning.

- Airways are more sensitive at night, and cold air may irritate sensitive airways.
- There may be a delayed response to an allergen to which the patient was exposed earlier.
- Postnasal drip or gastroesophageal reflux may occur because of sleeping position.

Gastroesophageal Reflux

Gastroesophageal reflux usually occurs at night, since the position we sleep in allows liquid to go the wrong way. When acid from the stomach leaks into the esophagus, most people experience heartburn. But if you have asthma, the backed-up acid from gastroesophageal reflux can lead to coughing and bronchospasm. Not eating for at least three hours before bedtime and sleeping with an extra pillow propped under the head helps many people; others require preventive medication to control the reflux, allowing them to get a good night's sleep.

Nasal Inflammation

The chronic nasal inflammation of sinusitis is one more common trigger of asthma. Sinusitis is an inflammation or infection of the sinus cavities, which open into the nasal passages. When the linings of the sinus passages become inflamed, mucus production increases and the sinuses cannot drain normally. Postnasal drip and a mild sore throat may result from nasal drainage, and drainage may lead to increased inflammation and twitchiness of the bronchioles. For people who experience sinus inflammation as well as asthma, identifying and controlling sinusitis can be the key to successful asthma management.

Strong Emotions

Powerful emotions, such as anger and fear, can lead to changes in breathing. Rapid, shallow breathing, or hyperventilation, can cause sensitive bronchial tubes to constrict, triggering the symptoms of asthma. Strong emotions can also worsen asthma symptoms in susceptible individuals.

An asthmatic person's best bet when symptoms occur is to keep calm and manage them; panic gets in the way and more severe bronchospasm may result. As we mentioned earlier, this does *not* mean that asthma is a psychosomatic disease. No degree of emotion can bring on asthma if you do not already have the hyperreactive airways that characterize this condition.

Cold Air and Other Changes in the Weather

Asthma symptoms can be worsened by climate, although climate affects people in different ways. The humidity of rainy days may bother some asthma sufferers; hot, dry weather can irritate the airways of others. Cold air, as we mentioned when we talked about exercise, can act on the sensitive airways of some asthmatics and cause symptoms. But others with asthma are overjoyed at the approach of winter—these asthmatics may suffer from seasonal allergies in the spring or fall.

Airborne Irritants

Many airborne irritants can inflame asthmatic airways and cause the muscles surrounding them to contract, bringing on the symptoms of asthma. The action of irritants in this process does not involve the production of the antibody IgE in an allergic reaction. In this case the harsh irritants themselves act on the airways.

Cigarette smoke is probably the greatest offender, but air pollutants such as ozone and sulfur dioxide are a growing problem. Aerosol sprays, cleaning products, gasoline fumes, industrial chemicals, paints, perfumes, and smoke from wood-burning stoves or burning leaves can all provoke asthma.

Secondhand Cigarette Smoke

A special note about the dangers of secondhand smoke: We have long known that inhaling cigarette smoke is hazardous to your health. Today there is a growing awareness that breathing in secondhand cigarette smoke also increases your risk of disease. Exposure to secondhand smoke is an especially sad situation for young children, who have no choice in the matter.

Studies show that children who live in homes with one or more smokers have more respiratory infections than do children who live in smoke-free environments. Maternal cigarette smoking can actually *double* a young child's risk of developing asthma, according to a study conducted by Scott T. Weiss, M.D., Ph.D., associate professor of medicine at the Harvard Medical School.

Children are most likely to develop asthma in response to smoking when they are exposed to secondhand smoke before the age of three. Although passive smoking does not seem to *cause* asthma in children over three, it can still *worsen* the symptoms of asthma in children who already have it. There is no reason to tolerate anyone's smoking around your child. Make your home a smoke-free zone.

Occupational Hazards

Occupational hazards, such as exposure to the chemicals used in the manufacture of glues, paints, plastics, and polyurethane foam, are another trigger of asthma. More than 200 chemicals have been shown to bring on symptoms. Often chemicals act as sensitizers, stimulating the production of the antibody IgE and introducing allergic reactions into the airways. Still, you don't need to have allergies or be allergy-prone to react to occupational hazards. Many chemicals are harsh irritants that can send the sensitive airways of asthmatics into bronchospasm. The best way to control occupational asthma is to remove yourself from exposure to the chemical that causes it.

Aspirin and Other Medications

When you have asthma it's especially important to monitor all medications that you take, whether they are prescription or over-the-counter. Be certain to speak to the physician treating your asthma whenever you want or need to incorporate a new medication into your medical regimen. There are three types of drugs that are generally not recommended for people who have asthma: aspirin and aspirin-like medications, beta-blockers, and sedatives. Whenever you are in doubt about taking a medication, consult your asthma doctor.

Aspirin

Aspirin and other nonsteroidal anti-inflammatory drugs (NSAIDs) are a trigger for as many as half of all asthma sufferers. People for whom aspirin is the primary trigger of asthma tend to be nonallergic and over the age of thirty. The reaction of asthmatics to aspirin is called idiosyncratic. This is because the exact mechanism by which aspirin triggers asthma symptoms is not known; it's not an allergic response, since there is no IgE antibody to aspirin.

Most asthma specialists recommend that aspirin and products that contain aspirin should simply be avoided by asthmatics, since acetaminophen products, such as Tylenol and Datril, are safe and widely available alternatives. If you are sensitive to aspirin, you should also steer clear of ibuprofen. Sold under the brand names Advil, Motrin, and Nuprin, ibuprofen is used like aspirin to relieve headaches, fever, and the joint pain of arthritis.

It is especially important to avoid aspirin and aspirin products if you have nasal polyps in addition to asthma. A condition known as triad asthma is a combination of asthma, nasal polyps, and aspirin sensitivity. The association of aspirin and nasal polyps can bring on sudden and severe breathing problems.

Beta-Blockers

Beta-blockers are commonly used to treat heart disease and high blood pressure, but beware: these drugs can also trigger asthma symptoms. Because beta-blockers may increase the level of muscle tone in airways, asthmatics may experience symptoms such as a tight chest or wheezing as a result of taking them. Even the use of eye drops containing beta-blocker medication can result in an asthma flare-up. Consult your doctor about alternative medications.

Tranquilizers

One of the biggest mistakes an asthmatic person can make is to take a tranquilizer, or sedative. Tranquilizers are often taken or administered with the best of intentions; parents have been known to give tranquilizers to their children to calm them down during or after an asthma attack. But tranquilizers have an extremely dangerous effect on asthmatics: tranquilizers sedate you and reduce your breathing capacity. In some cases of asthma, tranquilizers have caused death. During an asthma attack, it's important to stay awake, stay calm, and focus on your breathing. *Don't* take a tranquilizer.

Foods and Food Additives

A small percentage of people with asthma develop symptoms when exposed to certain foods or additives in processed foods. Some problem foods associated with asthma are shrimp, peanuts and other nuts, dairy products, and wheat. Food as a trigger is most common in children under five. If you suspect that food is a trigger for your child's asthma, you may want to see a board-certified allergist. Once you have identified the problem foods or food additives, eliminate them from your child's diet.

Some asthmatics should also steer clear of sulfites, which are frequently used to preserve food and to keep fruits and vegetables looking fresh. Metabisulfite (sodium bisulfite), one common food preservative and asthma trigger, can be found in cheese, wine, beer, sausage, pickles, and a variety of other fresh and processed foods. Sulfites unfortunately turn up in some medications as well.

Food additives too may be a problem for people with asthma. If you are sensitive to aspirin, it may be necessary to avoid Yellow Food Dye No. 5 (tartrazine), which is found in soft drinks, potato chips, candy, baked goods, pudding, cake mixes, and many other processed foods. The effect of Yellow Food Dye No. 5 on asthmatics seems to mimic that of aspirin in certain individuals. As with aspirin, the reaction of asthmatics to Yellow Food Dye No. 5 is called idiosyncratic, because the exact mechanism by which the dye triggers asthma symptoms is not known.

If you are sensitive to food preservatives or additives, carefully read labels and avoid foods, beverages, and medications that contain them. When in doubt, consult with your grocer or pharmacist. In restaurants, be sure to ask whether sulfites have been used at any point in the preparation of food.

CHAPTER 4

Making the Diagnosis and Working with Your Doctor

When wheezing, breathlessness, coughing, or other symptoms lead you to believe you have asthma, a careful and objective diagnosis should be your priority. If it is determined that asthma is the problem, your doctor can devise an appropriate medical regimen for the regular prevention and treatment of your symptoms.

It's important to remember that asthma is a chronic disease—not one that can be cured, but one that you may have to cope with again and again over the course of your lifetime. For this reason, it's crucial that you find a physician with whom you feel very comfortable, psychologically as well as on the basis of the doctor's expertise. You and the right doctor, working together as a team, can successfully manage this disease.

The Diagnosis of Asthma

The first step toward an accurate diagnosis of asthma includes a medical history and a thorough physical examination. Your personal medical history is of particular importance, since linking triggers and symptoms is a vital part of achieving control of your asthma.

Another important aspect of diagnosis involves objective measurement of lung function. Assessments of breathing called spirometry or pulmonary function tests measure the level of airflow obstruction in the lungs. Spirometry is often conducted as part of the examination of all patients suspected of having asthma.

A good working relationship with your doctor—one that stresses effective communication and mutual trust—is important throughout the process of asthma diagnosis and treatment. Be open and honest about behavior that may lead to asthma, such as smoking. Remember that your doctor is there to help you, not to judge you. If smoking is a problem, your physician can help you explore ways to quit. If exercise is a trigger for your asthma, a specialist can devise an aggressive medication program that will allow you to continue your exercise of choice.

Doctors look at many factors when diagnosing asthma. Diagnostic measures your doctor takes may include the following.

Your Medical History

Your doctor will take a thorough medical history before conducting a physical examination. An in-depth medical history is a key element of diagnosis. Again, it's essential that you trust your doctor: you should feel comfortable answering questions that will help your doctor diagnose and manage your asthma, just as he or she should be available to answer your questions about asthma.

Your doctor will ask you detailed questions concerning the presence of nighttime asthma, exercise-induced asthma, and absences from work and school. If you smoke, it's important to tell your doctor. Also let your doctor know about all drugs you take. Remember that your doctor can best diagnose and treat asthma if he or she has complete knowledge of your activities and symptoms.

If the initial medical history does not detect a pattern of triggers and symptoms, your doctor may recommend that you begin to keep a diary of your movements and symptoms. This more detailed record may provide clues. Remember too that family history is a vital part of your medical history; if you have a family member with asthma—especially a parent—you are much more likely to develop the condition.

A Thorough Physical Examination

A complete physical is the second step toward the diagnosis of asthma. Your height, weight, and blood pressure are usually taken first. Then your doctor will use a stethoscope to listen to your lungs. Since asthma reduces air flow through the lungs, your breathing rate can be a valuable sign as to whether or not you have asthma. Examination of the ears, nose, and throat is also important, since problems often occur in these, your upper airways, when you have asthma.

Breathing Tests

Your physician will take breathing tests to measure the level of obstruction in your airways. These tests, which are also known as spirometry or pulmonary function tests, are particularly important diagnostic tools. Breathing tests are an *objective* measure of lung function; subjective measures, such as physical examinations and medical histories, do not always accurately reflect the level of airway obstruction.

Spirometry can usually be conducted in your doctor's office. Doctors use an instrument called a spirometer to obtain such objective measurements as your:

- Peak expiratory flow rate (PEFR): the maximum flow rate of air in a forced exhalation from fully inflated lungs, as measured in either liters per second or liters per minute.
- Forced vital capacity (FVC): the total volume of air exhaled as rapidly and as long as possible.
- Forced expiratory volume 1 second (FEV1): the volume of air exhaled in one second from fully inflated lungs.
- Maximum midexpiratory flow rate (MMEF): the flow rate between 25 and 75 percent of the volume of a forced exhalation.

Although these breathing tests may appear somewhat complicated to asthma patients, they are actually the simplest and most effective tools your doctor has for diagnosing and evaluating asthma. If your doctor finds that you do indeed have asthma, he or she will show you how to use your own peak-flow meter to measure PEFR. A peak-flow meter is an inexpensive, hand-held device, which your doctor may ask you to use daily—usually once in the morning and once in the evening—to monitor how well your lungs are working.

Chest X Ray

Sometimes the thickening of bronchial walls—which is caused by the inflammation that characterizes asthma—can be detected in a chest X ray. Otherwise, although chest X rays are usually normal for asthmatics, doctors find them a helpful diagnostic tool in ruling out disorders that mimic asthma.

Chest X rays may identify alternative causes of breathlessness, wheezing, and coughing, such as heart disease, pneumonia, or the presence of a foreign body obstructing the airway. If you are pregnant or think you may be, inform your physician; the X ray will still be taken if necessary, but your womb will be shielded.

Sinus X Ray or CAT Scan

Inflammation of the sinuses is a common trigger of asthma symptoms. If your doctor suspects that the inflammation caused by a sinus disease is a trigger or complication of your asthma, diagnostic measures can be taken. Inflammation can often be detected by means of an X ray. Even more sensitive is a CAT scan (computerized axial tomography scan) of the sinuses, which is more accurate than a sinus X ray in diagnosing sinus disease.

Bronchial Provocation Testing

When the diagnosis of asthma is uncertain, your doctor may refer you to a specialist to perform bronchial provocation testing, also known as a bronchial or methacholine challenge.

A bronchial challenge is done when you are free of symptoms, so that the doctor can get a baseline measurement of your normal breathing and determine your reaction when suspected irritants are introduced. In this highly sensitive test, you will be instructed to inhale a very diluted solution of a suspected trigger. If the substance is indeed a trigger for your asthma, airways will constrict and mast cells will release histamine, resulting in symptoms.

The bronchial challenge is an extremely accurate indicator of airway hyperreactivity, which is the hallmark of asthma. But because bronchial provocation testing may produce serious reactions, it should only be done in a controlled setting under the supervision of an asthma specialist. The bronchial challenge is also a very expensive test, and is most commonly administered when occupational asthma is suspected or when the diagnosis of asthma is being questioned.

Exercise Challenge

If exercise is a suspected trigger of your asthma, your doctor may conduct an exercise challenge. An exercise challenge often consists of a brief period of time bicycling or running; your physician will conduct a test before and after exercise to assess your pulmonary function. An exercise challenge is relatively inexpensive in comparison to bronchial provocation testing. If exercise does prove to be a trigger, the challenge can also help your doctor determine the type and amount of medication you should take before exercise to block symptoms.

Exercise is extremely important for your overall health. As well as strengthening your lungs and heart, exercise contributes to your psychological well-being. If exercise is a trigger for your asthma, it does *not* mean you should stop exercising. It does mean that you have to take medication before or after you exercise. (Read more about asthma and exercise in Chapter 9.)

Allergy Testing

If your doctor suspects that allergies lie at the root of your asthma, you will probably be referred to an allergist for further tests. Like your regular physician, the allergist will take a detailed medical history and conduct a physical examination, but in this case the focus will be on allergies as well as asthma.

A good history of your activities and symptoms is often the key to identifying allergies. An allergist can zero in on the substances that most commonly provoke your asthmatic episodes, especially airborne allergens (animal dander and dust mites, pollen, mold spores, cigarette smoke, pollution, etc.).

Very often an allergist will discover the allergens that trigger your symptoms through your medical history and physical examination. When these alone are insufficient for diagnosis, or when your physician wants to verify that certain allergens are a problem, additional methods may be used. These often include:

- **Skin tests.** A skin test is the most common way in which allergists determine allergies. Skin testing is most useful in young asthmatics, for whom allergies are an especially common trigger. Although they are not as accurate in identifying food allergies, skin tests are very helpful in detecting allergies to pollens, molds, and environmental agents such as dust mites and animal dander.

The allergist conducts a skin test by pricking your arm or back with a needle and applying a diluted solution of a suspected allergen. The pinprick is tiny and not very painful. If you have an allergy to that substance, the skin around the pinprick will redden, and within minutes a small hive or welt will form. This means that IgE antibodies specific to the allergen are present and have responded by releasing histamine and other mediators from the mast cells. (Because the release of histamine is critical to this test, it will *not* be effective if you have taken an antihistamine.)

- **RAST tests.** The RAST (Radioallergosorbent Test) is a blood test that measures specific IgE antibodies in the blood against specific allergens. Its advantage over skin tests lies in the fact that only a single blood sample is required; the sample is sent to a central laboratory, and your doctor receives the results of the blood test after several weeks.

Yet many allergists continue to prefer skin tests over RAST tests. RAST tests are considerably more expensive than skin tests, the results take more time, and some questions linger concerning their accuracy. As these tests are refined, however, allergists may use them more frequently.

● **Elimination diets and challenge tests.** If foods or beverages—or the chemicals in them—are thought to trigger your asthma, your allergist may attempt an elimination diet to identify the culprits. Particular items may be eliminated on the basis of your medical history and food diary. If the allergist succeeds in identifying problem foods by using this technique, you should eliminate them from your diet permanently.

A challenge test involves gradually reintroducing eliminated foods—usually at the rate of one each week—into your diet. In a food challenge suspected allergens are often camouflaged; mixing them with other foods makes the identification process considerably more objective.

If you experience symptoms on the reintroduction of a food such as milk, eggs, or nuts, which are common allergens, your allergist has succeeded in confirming the identity of the food that triggers your symptoms. Since challenge tests do produce reactions to foods, they should not be used if your food sensitivity brings on severe or life-threatening symptoms. (Read about the role of diet in asthma in Chapter 10.)

Complete Blood Count

Some doctors also take a complete blood count (CBC) as part of the diagnosis of asthma. A laboratory test may reveal that the level of your white blood cells called eosinophils is higher than usual, which often happens when you experience asthma symptoms caused by an allergic response. A complete blood count, however, is not an essential diagnostic tool for asthma. In the vast majority of cases, the measures we described above are far more useful.

Managing the Three Types of Asthma

The National Institutes of Health has described three levels of asthma: mild, moderate, and severe. Each has its own general set of characteristics, and medical treatment is necessarily customized to the severity of each person's asthma. Keep in mind that everyone who has asthma—even if only a very mild case—should alert his or her physician to this fact. Aggressive management of asthma is the best way to keep your condition under control.

Mild Asthma

Mild asthma is characterized by brief and intermittent episodes of wheezing, coughing, or difficulty in breathing. Once or twice a month you may find that you wheeze or cough during the night. Between these episodes, you will probably experience no symptoms at all.

Inhaled beta-agonists are bronchodilators that can be used as needed to relieve mild symptoms of asthma. However, if you find that you are using these medications daily, inform your doctor. You may have moderate asthma, which calls for a more aggressive treatment program.

Moderate Asthma

Episodes of moderate asthma usually occur once or twice a week. You may experience nocturnal asthma, waking in the night, coughing, and wheezing. Exercise can also trigger moderate symptoms. In some cases, wheezing, coughing, and difficulty in breathing may last for several days at a time. Occasionally, you may require emergency care.

Anti-inflammatory medications are prescribed to prevent cases of moderate asthma, while inhaled beta-agonists are used to relieve symptoms when they do occur. An occasional short burst of oral corticosteroids may turn asthma around when your doctor is unable to control your condition with a combination of inhaled anti-inflammatory agents and bronchodilators.

Severe Asthma

If your asthma symptoms are continuous, or if you experience frequent attacks, you probably have severe asthma. Severe asthma can affect your overall level of activity and cause frequent nighttime symptoms. You may require hospitalization or occasional emergency treatment.

If you have severe asthma, you should be under the care of a specialist. Severe asthma often requires long-term treatment with oral corticosteroids; your specialist will closely monitor you for the potentially adverse side effects of this treatment program. (For more information on asthma medications, turn to Chapter 8.)

When to See an Asthma Specialist

There are times when it becomes necessary to reach beyond the care of your regular family internist, general practitioner, or pediatrician to enlist the expertise of an asthma specialist. An asthma specialist can be either an allergist or a pulmonologist.

We recommend that you seek the care of a specialist under the following circumstances:

- If you experience a life-threatening asthma attack.
- If you have sinusitis, nasal polyps, or vocal cord syndrome in addition to asthma.
- If occupational exposure is a complication of your asthma.
- If your routine treatment includes oral corticosteroids.
- If you require specific diagnostic tests.
- If you need further guidance or education to control your environment, to quit smoking, or to cope with complications of asthma treatment.
- If, despite treatment by your primary-care physician, you continue to experience nighttime asthma, find that you are missing work or school, are forced to curtail your desired exercise, or suffer side effects from medication.

Monitoring Your Asthma

Self-management is one of the most important techniques you can learn in the treatment of asthma. You can come to recognize the early-warning signs of your asthmatic episodes, and take medication to ward them off. If you see that your lung function is less than your personal best, temporarily increase your medication, according to your doctor's directions. Removing yourself from exposure to triggers is, of course, the right thing to do in virtually all circumstances.

There are two major strategies to follow in monitoring your asthma: learn to recognize the warning signs of your asthma, and use a peak-flow meter to objectively measure your lung function.

Recognizing the Warning Signs

While asthma attacks can be very frightening—especially when you experience the first one—in time you will see that there is a pattern to the clues that precede your episodes. Once you recognize the warning signs of an asthma attack, you can take medication to prevent it.

You already know that a substance or activity that is a potent trigger for one asthmatic may have no effect at all on another; likewise, the signals of an asthma attack differ from person to person. Learn to recognize which warning signs are important to you. The most common early-warning signs of asthma attacks are:

- Changes in breathing
- Sneezing
- Moodiness
- Headache
- A runny or stuffy nose
- A cough
- An itchy throat or chin

- Fatigue
- Dark circles under the eyes
- Insomnia

Using a Peak-Flow Meter

Virtually all asthmatics over the age of five can use a peak-flow meter to measure how well their lungs are working. If your doctor prescribes this relatively inexpensive device, your health insurance may cover all or part of its cost.

A peak-flow meter can provide an invaluable objective measurement of your peak expiratory flow rate, or PEFR. As we explained earlier in this chapter, PEFR is the maximum flow of air in a forced exhalation from fully inflated lungs, as measured in liters per second or per minute. Changes in this rate can alert you that an asthma attack will occur; you can then take medication to prevent it, as prescribed by your doctor.

When your asthma is moderate to severe, you should blow into your peak-flow meter twice each day, at about 7 A.M. and 7 P.M. (If you have a very mild case of asthma, taking PEFR measurements less frequently is okay.) Keep a record of your results and show them to your doctor, who can then determine the breathing rate that is normal for you, and what is your personal best.

Once your doctor has identified these breathing rates, and you feel comfortable using your peak-flow meter, you can objectively monitor your lung function—and therefore your asthma—every day. To help asthmatics use home PEFR monitoring, the National Institutes of

Health suggests a zone system that recalls a traffic light:

- Green Light (80 to 100 percent of your highest or personal best PEFR measurement): This means that asthma symptoms are not present and you should simply follow your routine treatment plan.
- Yellow Light (50 to 80 percent of your personal best): This often means that you are experiencing acute symptoms, in which case you require a temporary increase in medication. It can also indicate that chronic asthma is not sufficiently controlled, calling for an increase in maintenance medication.
- Red Light (50 percent or more below your personal best): This is the danger zone. A measurement this low means that you should immediately take bronchodilator medication. Notify your doctor if your PEFR measures do not return at once to the green or at least the yellow zone.

It's important to note that, useful as peak-flow meters are, many doctors prefer to stress a different style of patient education. Physicians can teach you as a patient to recognize an increase in symptoms, such as coughing or wheezing, as a guide to increasing your medication. You can then use a backup bronchodilator. If you find that you are using your backup medicine more frequently than every four hours, promptly contact the physician who is helping you manage your asthma.

Working with Your Doctor

The key to successful management of your asthma often lies in developing a good working relationship with your doctor. Besides diagnosing your asthma, your physician will help you:

- Identify the triggers of your asthma and work with you to devise strategies to avoid them.
- Develop an individualized medication program to keep your asthma under control.
- Monitor your asthma, and teach you how to monitor your condition as well.
- Teach you how to gain control over your asthma instead of allowing asthma to control you.

It's important that you have trust and confidence in the doctor you choose to treat your asthma. There are emotional adjustments you need to make when coping with a chronic disease such as asthma, and the right doctor can ease your way through any necessary transitions. He or she can help you understand your condition and guide you in its management. Finding a skilled physician with whom you feel comfortable is fundamental to successful asthma management.

- Seek out a doctor who will set aside enough time to answer your questions.
- Make sure that your doctor is accessible in case of emergency.
- Ask your doctor to arm you with a complete plan of action: what to do if your peak-flow rate falls into the yellow zone, what to do if your PEFR plummets to the red danger zone, what to do if

you develop adverse reactions to medication. It helps to have this plan in writing.

The inability to breathe is enough to strike fear in anyone but knowing how to get your breathing back to normal can reduce or eliminate this fear. The best weapon you have against the panic or anxiety sometimes provoked by asthma is *understanding*. Your doctor can help you understand that asthma is a serious but *reversible* condition. As we explained above, you can learn how to monitor your own asthma. Today there are tools available that can prevent the frantic trips to the emergency room that characterized asthma just ten or so years ago. By using today's state-of-the-art management techniques and medications, you can live a normal life with asthma.

CHAPTER 5

Your Child and Asthma

In the not so distant past, asthma was thought of as an acute illness of weak or overly emotional children. Children were needlessly restricted in their activities, often barred from exercise and participation in sports. Frequently the only treatment children received was medication to relieve asthma attacks.

Today we know that, for children as well as adults, asthma is a manageable condition that can be treated over the long term. Treatment focuses on the elimination of triggers and the use of preventive medication. Still, asthma continues to be a potentially dangerous condition that must be taken very seriously.

Asthma affects about one in every ten children, according to the American Academy of Allergy and Immunology. It is the most common chronic illness of childhood and a leading cause of children's absenteeism from school and visits to the hospital. The child with asthma faces special concerns, both physically and emotionally. And, like most chronic diseases of childhood, asthma affects not only your child—it has an impact on the entire family.

The Special Concerns of Childhood Asthma

Asthma in children is not the same as asthma in adults. As a parent, you already know that anything that makes your child feel "different" is a source of concern—and asthma *will* require your child to make some lifestyle adjustments.

The treatment of asthma usually involves taking regular medication and visiting the doctor more frequently than other children. Acute episodes may even entail an occasional visit to the emergency room. There are special concerns at school as well: an asthmatic child may need to take medication before participating in sports, or make unscheduled trips to the nurse's office to relieve acute symptoms. Children with chronic, uncontrolled asthma can even experience delayed growth problems.

There are many things that you as a parent can do to smooth your child's path and help him or her cope with asthma. Your attitude toward your child's illness will be pivotal; children take their parents' lead and approach asthma from a similar viewpoint. Dealing with your child's asthma in a calm and matter-of-fact manner is usually the best way to help him or her feel comfortable with the condition. It's essential to make sure that the child is familiar with the routine treatment of his or her asthma.

The more you and your child know about the child's asthma, the better able you will be to control it. Once you understand asthma, there is no reason to fear the disease. You and your child can learn to recognize the warning signs of an asthma attack, taking precautions to prevent it or lessen its severity. Asthma specialists recommend that parents also team up with health care providers and school personnel to help their child understand and manage their asthma.

Children Have Small Airways

Many parents wonder why this lung disease affects so many children. A chief reason lies in a simple physiological fact: children have smaller airways than adults. As in an adult who has asthma, hyperreactive, or twitchy, airways in your asthmatic child respond to a trigger by contracting and becoming inflamed. But because the airways in the child's lungs are so much smaller than those in an adult, they become blocked or obstructed more easily. The narrow airways of children grow yet narrower as they constrict in response to a trigger, resulting in the symptoms of asthma.

The Symptoms of Asthma in Children

Although the symptoms of asthma vary according to the size and age of the child, a major sign that any child has asthma is wheezing during a respiratory illness. Coughing at night is another clue. Asthma symptoms in children are by no means limited, however, to wheezing and coughing. If you notice any of the symptoms we describe here in your child, it's time to visit the pediatrician and see whether asthma is the problem.

The narrow airways of the smallest children, infants and toddlers, are more susceptible to obstruction. For this reason the symptoms in this age group may be more pronounced. In a young child, asthma may appear as:

- Rapid and noisy breathing
- A chest that appears concave or sucked in
- Chest congestion

Parents on the lookout for signs of asthma in an older child may notice that the child tires easily. Perhaps your child is short of breath and has less stamina on the playground. Sometimes children cut back on activity to avoid fits of coughing and wheezing. Other children complain of a tight chest, or suffer from cold after cold. The most common symptoms of asthma in older children are:

- Coughing
- Wheezing
- Shortness of breath
- A feeling of tightness in the chest

Asthma Lookalikes

A number of childhood diseases can mimic the symptoms of asthma. Chronic wheezing during a respiratory illness, coughing at night, or shortness of breath when exercising usually means that a child has asthma. But these symptoms can also be caused by other problems that only look like asthma. Regular visits to the doctor during asthma episodes will provide the information necessary to make an accurate diagnosis. Several childhood problems commonly mistaken for asthma are discussed below.

Airway Obstruction

Foreign objects such as peas, peanuts, popcorn, and even Mommy's rings have been known to make their way into children's lungs. The obvious discomfort, coughing, and wheezing that result are often mistaken for asthma. The key to diagnosis lies in the fact that an airway obstruction affects only one lung, while asthma affects both lungs. In children under two years of age, in whom foreign body aspirations are most apt to occur, diagnosis hinges on a careful history and a high index of suspicion.

Bronchiolitis

Bronchiolitis is an infection of the bronchioles, or small breathing tubes, in the lungs of infants. Bronchiolitis is almost always caused by a respiratory virus. Babies are susceptible to bronchiolitis because their airways are small and more easily blocked when infections occur. If your infant shows signs of difficulty in breathing, call your pediatrician immediately. Many infants who develop bronchiolitis develop asthma when they grow older.

Bronchitis

Bronchitis is an inflammation of the larger, more central breathing tubes in the lungs, and usually occurs as a complication of a viral respiratory illness. Bronchitis begins with a runny nose and difficult breathing, followed by a low-grade fever and cough. Mucus production is high. The child who suffers from recurrent bronchitis in most cases has asthma. If the illnesses are causing the child to miss school, referral to an asthma specialist is often warranted.

Croup

Croup is an inflammation of the larynx and trachea that makes breathing difficult. Infants and toddlers who have colds sometimes develop croup, which is characterized by a distinctive barking cough. Croup often comes on suddenly at night. Your child may suddenly experience difficulty in inhaling (as opposed to the difficulty in exhaling that characterizes asthma). If you suspect that your child has croup, get in touch at once with your pediatrician.

Cystic Fibrosis

Cystic fibrosis is an inherited childhood disease that affects the lungs and pancreas. Although progress has been made in its treatment, there is still no cure. A child with cystic fibrosis often has a persistent, asthma-like cough. Mucus in the lungs is thicker and more likely to become infected. Diagnosis of cystic fibrosis is made by measuring the amount of salt your child loses through perspiration.

Do Children Outgrow Asthma?

As children grow older, the airways in their lungs grow and the symptoms of asthma may gradually diminish and in many cases disappear. About half of all asthmatic children appear to outgrow asthma when they reach adolescence—but this does not mean that their airways are no longer hyperreactive, or twitchy. As airways grow larger and wider, muscle contraction does not result in the significant blockage that causes asthma symptoms.

Although children cannot outgrow asthma, they can outgrow some of its triggers. The triggers that set off asthma symptoms lessen with age. Asthma in children is often triggered by upper-respiratory infections and allergies, and these two problems frequently fade as children grow older.

For these reasons many children do appear to outgrow asthma. But it's important to remember that once a child has asthmatic airways, he or she has them for life. New triggers may set off the symptoms of asthma at any time, perhaps long after the child has passed into adulthood and years after the last asthmatic episode. The underlying condition of asthma remains the same; airways that are hyperreactive in a child continue to be hyperreactive as the child grows into adulthood.

The Triggers of Childhood Asthma

Heredity determines whether or not a child has the potential to develop asthma, but genetic predisposition alone does not cause asthma. Other factors play a role. The symptoms of asthma must be *triggered* by environmental stimulants.

Certain triggers have an especially strong impact on children. Experts agree that upper-respiratory infections are by far the most common trigger of asthma in children under five. Allergens, such as mold spores, pollen, and animal dander are also powerful triggers of asthma in children. Other common stimulants of asthma symptoms are irritants (such as cigarette, cigar, or pipe smoke), exercise, and cold air. Be certain you are aware of the triggers that bring on asthma symptoms in your child.

Upper-Respiratory Infections

The most common trigger of asthma in children is a viral respiratory infection. Infants and toddlers most often experience asthma symptoms related to conditions such as colds, bronchitis, croup, and the flu. Fortunately, as children grow older they contract fewer and fewer infections of this type.

Allergens

Asthma is closely linked with allergies in children. Asthma specialists estimate that up to 90 percent of children with asthma have allergies. In children, asthma can be considered an allergy of the lungs, much as hay fever is an allergy of the nose and throat.

Common allergens that provoke asthma symptoms are pets, mold spores, pollen, and house-dust mites (found in bedding, stuffed animals, and carpets). If you suspect that allergies lie at the root of your child's asthma, see a board-certified allergist to determine which allergens are the ones that affect your child. You can control your child's asthma by eliminating those allergens from your environment.

Irritants

Many substances in the environment can irritate your child's sensitive airways, even if your child is not actually allergic to them. Cigarette smoke is the most common irritant: *no one* should be allowed to smoke in the home of an asthmatic child. You may also want to eliminate other sources of strong odors (such as perfumes and aerosol sprays) from your home.

Exercise

We can't say it often enough: exercise is very important for asthmatics. Many Olympic athletes compete in spite of asthma. Exercise is good for a child's body and builds self-esteem. If exercise is a trigger for your child's asthma, ask your doctor about premedication. Inhaled medications such as cromolyn sodium can be used fifteen minutes before exercise to prevent symptoms from developing.

Avoiding the Triggers of Asthma

An important part of asthma management is identifying and removing the triggers of asthma from your child's environment. Medication is an essential part of the treatment plan, but it is no substitute for eliminating triggers whenever and wherever possible. If your child is allergic to house-dust mites or mold, for example, take measures to lessen exposure. If a much-beloved pet is the problem, limit contact. Following are some tips on avoiding the many triggers of asthma. (For an in-depth look at eliminating triggers, turn to Chapter 7.)

- Concentrate on your child's bedroom, where a third or more of the child's time is spent. Keep the bedroom as clean and dust-free as possible. Don't let a pet to which your child is sensitive enter the bedroom.
- Every week, wash all your child's bedding in very hot water (at least 130 degrees Fahrenheit).
- Cover your child's mattress, box spring, and pillow with airtight cases.
- Avoid feather pillows and blankets made from wool or down.
- Invest in an air purifier, or install a filter in your heating and air-conditioning systems.
- Keep your kitchen and bathroom well ventilated and free of mold.
- If you use a humidifier, clean it regularly to reduce the growth of mold and bacteria.
- Avoid sources of strong odors, such as cleaning fluids, aerosol sprays, and perfumes.
- *Don't smoke!* And don't allow anyone else in your

home to smoke. Cigarette smoke is a powerful trigger of asthma in children.

Asthma Medications for Children

Like adults, children take two types of medication to treat the symptoms of asthma: anti-inflammatories, which reduce inflammation and decrease mucus production, and bronchodilators, which relax muscles in the airway, and stop the spasms of an asthma attack. Depending on the nature of your child's asthma, medications will be prescribed to be taken regularly or as needed. Often doctors prescribe a combination of medications for children.

Children older than five or so take inhaled medications through metered-dose inhalers, also known as MDIs or puffers. Inhaling medication directly into the lungs has the advantage of working immediately on the airways, and because only minuscule amounts of inhaled drugs enter the bloodstream, they have fewer side effects. Children must be taught to use an MDI correctly to gain full benefit from it. A spacer device, available at most pharmacies, can be attached to the canister of the inhaler to ensure that the appropriate amount of medication reaches the child's lungs.

Because very young children may have difficulty manipulating metered-dose inhalers, doctors often recommend that preschoolers instead use devices called nebulizers. These are small electric or battery-run machines that spray medication directly into a child's airways via a mask placed over the nose and mouth.

The medication prescribed for your child will depend on the nature of your child's asthma:

- If your child's asthma is chronic and disrupts day-to-day life, your pediatrician will probably prescribe preventive anti-inflammatory medications. These include cromolyn sodium and inhaled steroids. Because these drugs are preventive, it's especially important to take them regularly, as directed by the doctor. The child should not skip doses or stop taking medication because symptoms subside.

- Bronchodilators are the drugs of choice for the relief of acute asthma attacks. Beta-agonists and other bronchodilators act to relax muscles and open airways. Bronchodilators are used in inhaled form for the relief of asthma attacks; controlled-release pills are recommended for maintenance therapy in severe cases of asthma.

When It's Time to See a Specialist

Many times a child's asthma requires treatment above and beyond that provided by your regular pediatrician. When consulting a physician who specializes in treating asthma, you may choose to see either an allergist or a pulmonologist.

We recommend that you seek the care of a specialist under the following circumstances:

- If your child experiences a life-threatening asthma attack.
- If your child has sinusitis, nasal polyps, or vocal cord syndrome in addition to asthma.
- If your child is taking oral corticosteroids regularly.

- If your child requires specific diagnostic tests.
- If your child needs more thorough asthma education and guidance in self-management techniques.
- If, despite the pediatrician's treatment, your child continues to experience nighttime asthma, is missing school, cannot perform desired exercise, or is suffering side effects of medication.

The Impact of Asthma on Children

Children with mild, well-controlled asthma suffer few physical or emotional consequences. Severe or poorly controlled asthma, on the other hand, can lead to problems. A small number of children may encounter physical or psychological difficulties caused by asthma.

Physical Consequences

Again, most children do not experience any serious physical repercussions from asthma. But if a child's asthma is very serious or inadequately controlled, he or she may fail to thrive. Especially when oral steroids are used in the treatment of asthma, a child's growth can be stunted. Because of this, long-term use of oral steroids is not recommended in most cases, and any child who appears to need this type of treatment should be under the care of an asthma specialist.

Although bronchodilators are used to relieve asthma attacks, asthma specialists warn against "bronchodilator abuse." This is an overuse of bronchodilators, a sign that asthma is poorly controlled. If your child regularly needs to use beta-agonists more than twice a day, the

symptoms are being relieved while the underlying inflammation in the lungs may be worsening. Eventually
this situation can prove life-threatening. In this case
your child's treatment should be corrected to include
anti-inflammatories, which reduce and prevent inflammation in the airways.

Psychological Consequences

Although asthma is brought on by sensitive
airways—and is NOT psychosomatic—the condition can
generate a confusing whirlpool of emotions in some children. Children have been known to feel anger, fear, de-
pression, loneliness, guilt, and inferiority in response to
asthma.

Children tend to have troubling feelings when their
asthma is not well managed. If a child has felt angry
and fearful when rushed to the emergency room during
an asthma attack, make sure that next time the child
understands exactly what is happening. Be very clear
about the treatment plan, and invite the child to participate in that plan as fully as his or her age allows. Encourage him or her to think positively: the asthma can
be handled. Once your child feels more control over
asthma, he or she will be less likely to experience negative psychological consequences from it.

The Impact of Asthma on the Family

Like other chronic childhood diseases, asthma affects not just the child but the whole family. Parents may be reluctant to discipline a child with asthma for fear of provoking an attack, and this reluctance can lead to difficult interactions throughout the family. Other children may resent the "favored" child, while the asthmatic child fails to learn the consistent structure and limits all children need.

Sometimes outside counseling becomes advisable for a child. A depressed teenager may ignore the warning signs of an asthma attack, or skip medication. Other children may use asthma to avoid school or to manipulate the family.

Asthma may sometimes exaggerate problems that already exist in the family, and children from unstable homes have been shown to be more susceptible to asthma attacks. In these cases family counseling can help.

Parents under pressure can always seek the relief of other family members, friends, clergy, or professional counselors. There are also many organizations that provide support for parents of asthmatics. Mothers of Asthmatics, for example, has a network of local support groups and provides addresses of summer camps for asthmatic children. (Turn to Chapter 12 for more information on asthma resources.)

Asthma at School

Children need to learn how to control their asthma away from home, especially at school, where they spend so much time. Some children fall behind in their school-work if they miss class time because of asthma. Yet although severe asthma may call for hospitalization, a mild episode of asthma can be handled at school. A few minutes in the nurse's office are usually all that's necessary to relieve the symptoms of the asthma sufferers, after which the child can quickly return to the classroom or athletic field. This is a far cry from the time when an asthma attack would automatically require a trip to the emergency room.

It's vital that parents of asthmatic children keep an open line of communication with all school personnel directly concerned with the child, especially the teacher, school nurse, and principal. The American Academy of Allergy and Immunology recommends that parents prepare for school by doing the following:

- Check the classroom to make sure it doesn't contain substances that trigger your child's asthma. If you find an old rug or moldy floor, which may set off symptoms in your child, ask whether it can be removed, or request that your child be moved to a different classroom.

- Schedule a conference before the start of the school year so that involved personnel will understand your child's asthma. Explain the triggers of your child's asthma. Ask questions about the curriculum. Art projects, for example, may involve paint and glue, possible triggers. Other classrooms might have pets to which your child is sensitive.

- Make sure your child's teacher understands what to do if symptoms develop. Explain what medications your child takes and what side effects, if any, to expect from them.

• Emphasize the importance to your child of physical education. If premedication is necessary for your child to participate in exercise, inform the school nurse and the physical education teacher.

• Encourage your child's teacher to adopt the same efficient yet matter-of-fact attitude about your child's asthma that you have. The consistency of approach will help your child smoothly adjust to school, and not make him or her feel "different" from other children.

• File a written treatment plan with your school. Ask your doctor to write down instructions for your child's medication and where to seek emergency care (your doctor's office or the emergency room of a nearby hospital) if your child does not respond to treatment.

Summer Camps for Asthmatic Children

Asthma is a fairly common childhood problem, and many established summer camps have very good facilities for coping with asthmatic children. Still, parents of asthmatic children often prefer to send their children to summer camps specifically designed to meet the needs of asthmatic children.

Summer camps for asthmatic children, which began to appear in the 1950s, provide expert medical supervision in an atmosphere that encourages asthmatics to enjoy a wide range of physical activities. A child whose asthma is well controlled should be able to run and play as hard as any other child.

Children are encouraged to take part in a wide range of outdoor activities, as at any summer camp. But they are also taught valuable techniques of asthma self-care. Children develop self-confidence as well as having a good time.

Asthma Management

With a good understanding of asthma and full use of the excellent medical care available today, you and your child can keep asthma under control. Self-care is the most valuable coping mechanism children can learn.

Pediatricians recommend that children as young as age four begin to use their own peak-flow meters each day to monitor asthma. These hand-held devices measure the volume and speed at which air can be expelled from the lungs, and can help predict when symptoms will occur.

Children can also learn which triggers bring on the symptoms of their asthma, and how to avoid them. They can come to recognize the warning signs of an asthma attack and take preventive medication. In fact, children should begin to participate in their medication program as soon as age and maturity allow.

Above all, you as a parent can project a positive attitude about asthma to your child, and encourage your child to approach asthma in a positive manner. Don't panic when your child has an asthma attack: have a written treatment plan from your doctor that outlines exactly what steps you should take. Many children in the United States have asthma, and there are numerous resources that parents can take advantage of to help children understand and manage the condition. Do your best to make sure that you and your child are as knowledgeable and confident as possible in the management of asthma.

CHAPTER 6

Asthma and Special Situations

Some additional thought must be given to coping with asthma when unusual situations arise. Special events—situations which take us out of our everyday way of living—are part of most lives. Women with asthma become mothers; many of us undergo surgical procedures; and we work, sometimes in environments in which we are unfortunately exposed to harmful chemicals or pollutants.

Everyone must take extra care and make additional preparations when significant changes in lifestyle occur. If you have asthma, even more complicated arrangements are usually necessary. In most cases, there are specific steps you can take to control your asthma, minimizing its impact on your life during events such as pregnancy and surgery.

When asthma is effectively managed by you and your physician, you can weather changes in your life. With proper care, you can continue to function normally, without aggravating the symptoms of your asthma, as you pass through the stages of your life.

Asthma and Pregnancy

As many as 4 in every 100 women experience asthma symptoms during pregnancy. Pregnancy and childbirth are special times in a woman's life, yet women who have asthma are often anxious about the impact asthma will have on the pregnancy. Important questions arise: What effect does asthma medication have on an unborn child? And what happens to the health of both mother and child if asthma is left untreated during pregnancy?

The best medical answer available today lies in a balanced approach to asthma and pregnancy. Asthma management is basically comprised of two elements: avoiding triggers that provoke symptoms, and using medication to prevent symptoms or to relieve them if they do occur. Avoiding triggers is especially important during pregnancy, in order to reduce the need for medication. Certain medications are considered safe to use during pregnancy; others are not recommended.

The bottom line is that, with appropriate management, mothers with asthma can have normal pregnancies and healthy babies. There is no question that having asthma adds a very serious dimension to pregnancy; it's essential to control asthma in pregnant patients, and both your obstetrician and asthma specialist should be involved in treatment. But when asthma is well monitored and well controlled, there should be no adverse effect on either mother or baby.

Avoiding Triggers During Pregnancy

Avoiding triggers is the first line of defense against asthma attacks and can also reduce your need for medication during pregnancy. If you smoke, the best thing you can do for yourself and your baby is to quit today; not only does smoking worsen asthma, it can cause serious harm to your unborn baby.

We recommend that pregnant women take the following measures to avoid exposure to asthma-inducing allergens:

- Remove pets from the household, or at least ban them from your bedroom.
- Encase bedding in airtight covers.
- Wash bedding weekly in very hot water.
- Keep the humidity in your home below 50 percent.
- While frequent vacuuming is necessary, vacuuming raises dust. Ask someone else to do it, or wear a mask.
- In pollen season, close the windows and use air-conditioning.
- Avoid vigorous outdoor activity early in the morning, when pollen counts are highest.

Taking Medication While Pregnant

All things being equal, it's preferable not to take medication during pregnancy. But all things are not equal if you have asthma. The need for medication to prevent and relieve symptoms must be carefully weighed against the very serious health risks that may be posed by uncontrolled asthma. Poorly controlled asthma can lead to premature births, low birth weight, and even miscarriage, according to the National Institutes of Health.

The majority of women who must take medication for asthma before pregnancy will continue to require medication while pregnant. But which asthma medications are the safest for use by pregnant women?

Medications that have been shown to be safe for use during pregnancy are:

- Inhaled bronchodilators, such as terbutaline and albuterol
- Oral bronchodilators, such as theophylline
- Inhaled anti-inflammatory agents, such as cromolyn sodium and beclomethasone

Oral prednisone is also safe to use when it is necessary to control a pregnant woman's asthma. Epinephrine can be used in an emergency but Sus-phrine (a long-acting form of epinephrine) should be avoided.

Many pregnant women are already being treated with immunotherapy, or allergy shots, to control their allergies. Immunotherapy can safely be continued during pregnancy; in fact, its continued use during pregnancy may mean that less medicine will be required to control symptoms. Skin testing, on the other hand, should be avoided during pregnancy, as should increases in immunotherapy concentrations.

If you have asthma, you may also suffer from occasional allergic nasal symptoms. To relieve this discomfort during pregnancy, antihistamines such as chlorpheniramine and tripelennamine are considered safe. Loratadine, a new nonsedating antihistamine, may also be safe to use during pregnancy, although studies confirming its safety are not yet available. If necessary, intranasal cromolyn or beclomethasone can also be taken to control nasal symptoms.

Drugs occasionally used for treating asthma or nasal problems that should be avoided during pregnancy include:

- Antihistamines other than chlorpheniramine and tripelennamine
- Iodides
- Pseudoephedrine
- Sulfa antibiotics
- Tetracycline

Just as you would not expect your asthma doctor to help you give birth to your baby, you should not expect your obstetrician or midwife to manage your asthma.

Surgery and Asthma

Because surgery involves anesthesia and reduces respiratory capacity, an asthmatic patient undergoing a surgical procedure can face some additional risk. It's extremely important that you inform both your surgeon and the anesthesiologist that you have asthma, even if your asthma is very mild or if you have not experienced symptoms for some time. Likewise, the doctor responsible for treating your asthma must be informed that you plan to undergo surgery so that he or she can take appropriate measures to optimize your lung function before surgery. With careful planning and effective communication among your physicians, the risk of surgical complications caused by asthma can be held to a minimum.

Preparing Yourself for Surgery

Fear or anger can cause hyperventilation and provoke asthma symptoms; anxiety about a surgical procedure can prompt your twitchy airways to lapse right into bronchospasm. As you know by now, the best way to cope with your asthma is to thoroughly understand and manage it; this is also a good approach to surgery, as well as to any other physical ailment or procedure.

Talk to your surgeon, or to another health professional in the office if the surgeon is not available. Explain that you want to know exactly what is going to happen in surgery and why. Ask questions about how you should expect to feel afterward, and inquire about possible risks. If there are options for the type of anesthesia you will be given, make it clear that you want to be involved in the choice. Asking and getting answers to questions like these will remove the fear you may have of the unknown.

Medical Preparation for Surgery

If you have asthma and require surgery, you need three doctors: the surgeon, the anesthesiologist, and the doctor who regularly treats your asthma. It's essential that your asthma doctor obtain an objective measure of your lung function before surgery; this can usually be done in the doctor's office, through spirometry. (Turn to Chapter 4 for an explanation of this procedure.) Your doctor can then act to maximize your lung function before surgery. He or she can also discuss with the anesthesiologist the type of anesthesia that is most appropriate for you.

If you are taking oral corticosteroids, your asthma doctor will prescribe additional amounts of these drugs before surgery. You may not be able to take oral medication for some time after extensive surgery, so additional corticosteroids are necessary to prevent a potentially dangerous asthma attack.

Be certain that you inform your physicians of all the drugs you are taking. Many drugs can have dangerous interactions with anesthetics and other medications used during surgery. Don't neglect to mention over-the-counter medications; these are often very potent drugs. Aspirin and other NSAIDs, for example, should not be used in the period surrounding surgery, since they can promote bleeding. Also inform your physicians of any drugs you have taken that are not legal. Remember that all information is confidential, and the doctors treating you must have all the facts to care for you most effectively.

Anesthesia and Surgery

There are three types of anesthesia: local, spinal, and general. It's sometimes possible for the patient to voice an opinion favoring a certain type of anesthesia, but often the surgical procedure itself determines that general anesthesia is appropriate. The most important thing to do is let the anesthesiologist know that you have asthma.

Local and spinal anesthesia have often been considered better options than general anesthesia for asthmatics, since they numb the nerves that affect the surgical area but do not affect breathing. General anesthesia, on the other hand, entails loss of consciousness, during which breathing must be controlled by the anesthesiologist. Fortunately, the general anesthetics used today are safe for the person whose asthma is well controlled.

- **Local Anesthesia.** Local anesthesia is injected directly into the area on which surgery is being performed. If you have asthma, this numbing procedure is often preferable to general anesthesia, since it allows you to continue breathing on your own.

Many types of surgery can be performed using only a local anesthetic. But be sure that your doctor—or dentist, since dentists often inject local anesthetics—is aware that you have asthma. If there is a possibility that you may be sensitive to a local anesthetic, discuss it. Alternative medications are always available.

- **Spinal Anesthesia.** In a spinal block, the anesthestic is injected into the spinal cord. This anesthetizes a local area, but allows the patient to remain awake and breathe on his or her own. Many women are familiar with "spinals," since they are often the anesthesia of choice in cesarean sections. Spinals are a good alternative for asthmatics since, like local anesthestics, they do not affect breathing.

- **General Anesthesia.** In general or pulmonary anesthesia, you gradually lose consciousness as you inhale gas through a mask. The anesthesiologist carefully monitors this process. Once you are unconscious, the anesthesiologist takes control of your breathing by placing a breathing tube in your airway. The anesthestic halothane and its derivatives, often used in general anesthesia, may be particularly beneficial to asthmatics, since they are bronchodilators.

Postsurgical Care

Some asthma medications—such as theophylline, which is usually taken orally—can be given intravenously after surgery.

Special treatment is also required if you take oral corticosteroids for your asthma. Normally your body responds to the stress of surgery by producing cortisone. But if you have been taking oral corticosteroids (the chemical equivalent of cortisone), your body may have lost the ability to produce cortisone on its own. Cortisone helps your body handle stress; a lack of it may have serious consequences, such as a drop in blood pressure. You should not be alarmed if your postsurgical care involves intravenous treatment with corticosteroids for several days. Other bronchodilator medication can be given by inhalation, using a nebulizer or metered-dose inhaler.

Emergency Surgery

The most serious surgical danger faced by asthmatics is probably emergency surgery. A car accident, for example, can send an asthmatic patient to the hospital with no opportunity to discuss his or her condition with doctors. For this reason, your doctor may recommend that you always wear a Medic Alert bracelet advising health workers of your condition. This is especially true for asthmatics who take oral corticosteroids regularly.

Occupational Asthma

About 2 percent of asthma cases are caused by exposure to job-related irritants. Substances at work can sensitize your airways, often triggering serious asthma attacks. Early diagnosis and treatment of occupational asthma are crucial. Once you have become sensitized, your lungs can go into bronchospasm with even minimal exposure to the trigger. Most importantly, occupational asthma—unlike most other forms of asthma—may not be completely reversible. Constant exposure to irritants can permanently damage your airways.

Allergy or Sensitivity?

The potential for a true allergic response is present after your body has been exposed to an allergen and has produced IgE antibodies, which have contact with the mast cells in your body. When the allergen reenters your system, your mast cells respond by releasing histamine, which brings on the symptoms of asthma. (In Chapter 3 we traced the course of an allergic reaction.)

If you experience symptoms because of exposure to chemicals, odors, or bacteria in your workplace, it does not necessarily follow that you are *allergic* to those substances. Your reaction may instead be the result of a *sensitivity* to an irritant, which is not an IgE-related or allergic response. Many strong odors can irritate the twitchy airways of an asthmatic and provoke symptoms.

Whether your reactions are caused by an allergy or irritation, the best thing you can do is to identify and avoid the offending substance.

Common Triggers of Occupational Asthma

There are many causes of occupational asthma. If you work outside, constant exposure to pollutants such as ozone and sulfur dioxide may trigger symptoms. People who have asthma should do their best to avoid working in the chemical or petrochemical industries, where they may be bombarded with the fumes of harsh chemicals. Then there is the case of "baker's asthma," in which bakers and flour-mill workers experience allergic symptoms when exposed to flours such as wheat or rye.

Industries commonly linked to occupation asthma include:

- Chemical
- Dye
- Farming
- Food processing
- Glue
- Metal refining
- Paint
- Petrochemical
- Pharmaceutical
- Plastic
- Polyurethane foam
- Printing
- Rubber
- Textile
- Woodworking

Occupational Asthma and Delayed Reactions

Sometimes asthma attacks occur immediately after exposure to an irritant in the workplace. In these cases of constricted airways, asthma can be treated with a bronchodilator. At other times, occupational asthma may be difficult to diagnose and treat, since it can be characterized by delayed reactions. Symptoms may appear four to six hours after exposure to a trigger, usually as a result of inflammation in the airways. In these cases, treatment with corticosteroids may be the temporary answer. But occupational asthma may eventually lead to irreversible airway damage, so often the best management lies in removing yourself from that workplace.

Management of Occupational Asthma

As we've mentioned, medication can be a big help in the treatment of occupational asthma. Your doctor may prescribe one or a combination of bronchodilators, theophylline, cromolyn, and corticosteroids to relieve and control your symptoms.

Yet beneficial as medications may be, avoidance is still the safest and most effective way to control occupational asthma. Relentless long-term exposure to triggers in your workplace can wear your lungs down, causing irreversible damage in your airways. This is an extremely serious and potentially life-threatening consequence. If your doctor has made a clear diagnosis of occupational asthma, the best thing you can do is remove yourself from your present work environment.

CHAPTER 7

Controlling Your Environment

Once you have identified the substances that trigger your asthma, it's time to make some changes in your environment in an effort to avoid them. In fact, identifying and avoiding triggers is the first line of defense against asthma attacks. Asthma experts have found that one of the best ways you can control your asthma is to exert control over your environment. When you minimize your exposure to the stimuli that induce asthma, you get the added benefit of reducing your need for medication.

There are many practical ways in which you can eliminate house-dust mites, mold growth, pollen, and other common triggers of asthma from your surroundings. If you smoke, it's time to quit. Do not allow anyone to smoke in your home, and make sure smoke-free zones are part of your work environment. You may also want to vacuum your house or apartment more frequently; ban the family pet from your bedroom; get somebody else to do asthma-inducing chores, such as mowing the lawn or painting the house, and go "green," replacing some of the many harsh chemicals you use in your day-to-day life with safe and natural alternatives.

In the Home

If you or someone you live with has asthma, it's important to keep your home as free as possible of house dust and dust mites, mold, smoke, animal dander, pollen, and chemical irritants. This can be quite a job, but the reward of breathing easy—in the most literal sense—is worth the time and trouble.

Eliminate Dust and Dust Mites

House dust is a mixture of organic and inorganic matter. It combines materials such as skin cells shed by people or pets, pollen, and tiny bits of food. It's not actually the dust to which asthmatic people are sensitive: it's the microscopic house-dust mites that thrive on that dust. Here are some ways to get rid of dust and dust mites:

- Thoroughly clean your house on a regular basis.
- Dust regularly with a damp cloth, which will remove dust rather than simply spread it around.
- Vaccum every week with a strong canister-style machine.
- If an expensive vacuum cleaner is out of the question, use high-efficiency dust bags. While they cost two or three times the amount of standard bags,

high-efficiency bags fit most upright and canister vacuum cleaners and contain electrostatically charged fibers that trap far more dust than do standard bags.

- Since vacuuming can raise a significant amount of dust and thus trigger asthma symptoms, try to enlist a friend or family member to do the job for you. If that proves impractical, wear a dust mask when you vacuum to minimize your exposure. Keep in mind that dust particles remain in the air for about an hour after vacuuming.
- Vaccum not only rugs, but also floors, upholstered furniture, curtains, and pillows.

Eliminate Dust-Collectors

If you have asthma, don't allow clutter to accumulate in your home. A home filled with fussy knickknacks is an invitation to dust. Try to keep your home clean and simple. Some strategies that can help include:

- Try not to decorate your home with too many elaborate furnishings and decorations.
- Don't use wall-to-wall carpeting. Clean wood or linoleum floors are the best way to asthma-proof your home. If rugs are a must, choose thickly woven throw rugs and launder them frequently.
- Replace heavy drapes with light and easier-to-clean curtains or venetian blinds.
- Be aware that simply painted walls are best. Wallpaper- and fabric-covered walls collect dust.

Clear the Air

Airborne irritants—especially house dust, mold spores, pollen, and animal dander—are among the most common triggers of asthma. When you breathe in these substances, your twitchy asthmatic airways may go into spasm, resulting in symptoms such as breathlessness, wheezing, coughing, and tight chest. To avoid airborne irritants:

- Stress to your family and friends that your home is a smoke-free environment. It is a well-known fact that smoking can aggravate asthma, especially in children.
- Install air-conditioning in your home to lessen exposure to allergens.
- Use an electrostatic filter in your air conditioner to remove pollutants from household air. Replace the filter regularly—otherwise, air conditioners will simply recirculate dust and other airborne irritants.
- Install an air filter or purifier to clean household air. The best filters use a High Efficiency Particle Accumulation (HEPA) system.
- Keep humidity in your home below 50 percent to stave off development of mold spores. You may need a dehumidifier in damp basements and bathrooms.
- Clean the collecting pans in your dehumidifiers regularly.
- If your asthma symptoms are seasonal, close the windows to avoid exposure to pollen and other airborne triggers. Use air-conditioning.
- Avoid using toxic chemical cleaners or pesticides

in your home. Their fumes may trigger asthma. (*Nontoxic, Natural, and Earthwise,* by Debra Lynn Dadd, published by Jeremy P. Tarcher in 1990, is a great source of products you can use instead of harsh and potentially asthma-provoking chemicals.)

- If your house needs a fresh coat of paint, hire someone else to do the job. The fumes from paint are a potential trigger.
- Avoid air fresheners and potpourri—their odors can trigger asthma.

In the Bedroom

People spend about a third of their lives in their bedrooms. If you are sensitive to dust and dust mites, the comfort of a good night's sleep in your bedroom may be replaced by a nightmare of wheezing and congestion. Asthma specialists underline the importance of removing all possible triggers of asthma from your bedroom.

Asthma-Proof Your Bed

Dust mites, a potent allergen and trigger of asthma, thrive on the skin cells you unwittingly shed on bedroom linens. They nest in warm, damp mattresses. Here are some tips to help you asthma-proof your bed:

- Use nonallergenic Dacron pillows, instead of pillows stuffed with down or feathers. Foam pillows are also out—they may grow moldy because of perspiration.

- Buy new pillows every year or two.
- Avoid blankets and quilts made from wool or down. Washable nylon blankets are a better alternative.
- Use undyed cotton sheets.
- Encase your mattress and pillows in airtight plastic or nylon covers. Place mattress pads over stiff or uncomfortable plastic covers.
- If they are not covered, vacuum your mattress and box spring weekly.
- Wash all bedding weekly in very hot (130 degrees Fahrenheit) water.
- Air out all bedding regularly.

Make Your Bedroom a Haven from Asthma

People with asthma who have taken measures to asthma-proof their bedrooms have reduced both asthma episodes and their need for medication. Make a special effort to asthma-proof your bedroom:

- Don't store anything under your bed.
- Make your bedroom out-of-bounds to furry or feathered household pets.
- Don't decorate your bedroom with dust-collecting knickknacks.
- Don't use potpourri. Attractive dried flowers may unfortunately contain asthma-inducing molds, and their odor may also bring on symptoms.
- Use plain wood furniture in place of upholstered pieces. Ornately carved furniture and canopy beds are dust-collectors.

- If you want bookshelves in your bedroom, get the kind with glass doors.
- Keep your bedroom closet clean and orderly. Keep the door closed and the clothes off the floor.
- Avoid using perfumes and other scented beauty products, which are sources of potent odors and therefore potential asthma triggers.
- If you can't afford air-conditioning throughout your house, try at least to invest in an air conditioner for your bedroom.
- During pollen season (if pollen is a problem for you), keep the windows closed and the air conditioner on.
- In your child's bedroom, try to limit stuffed animals to one hypoallergenic, machine-washable teddy bear or bunny.

In the Bathroom, Kitchen, and Basement

The bathroom is the most likely room in your home to be affected by mold, another common trigger of asthma. Although outdoor mold spores are seasonal, mold (also called mildew) can flourish year-round in moist and humid indoor spaces. It's important to keep the growth of mold spores under control in the bathroom, kitchen, and basement. Strong odors, another trigger of asthma, should be avoided throughout your home. Strategies to asthma-proof these areas include:

- Be sure that your bathroom, kitchen, and basement are properly ventilated.
- Avoid using scented cleaning products.

- Scrub shower curtains, bathroom tiles, and fixtures regularly. Don't neglect hard-to-reach corners, where mildew can flourish.
- When you clean, avoid using commercial products that are scented or have particularly strong odors. Instead use safe and natural cleaning substances, such as baking soda, distilled white vinegar, lemon juice, liquid soap, and borax.
- Keep your refrigerator clean and orderly. Promptly use leftovers and throw out spoiled foods.
- Repair leaky basements, an open invitation to mold growth.
- Install dehumidifiers where necessary.

Your Lawn and Garden

To an asthmatic who suffers from seasonal symptoms, stepping outside to get a breath of fresh air is a real problem at certain times of year. If you have asthma for which pollen is a trigger, be sure you know the seasonal pattern for your area. (Your local chapter of the American Lung Association is a convenient source of this information.) Pollens, mold, pollution, and pesticide residues are all potential triggers that you can encounter on your lawn or in your garden. Here are some strategies to avoid them:

- Keep an eye on the pollen count. The numbers themselves may not mean much to you—but when you read in the newspaper that the pollen count is down, it's probably safe to spend time outdoors. When the pollen count is up, exercise caution: stay inside, close the windows, and switch on the air conditioner.

- Avoid engaging in strenuous outdoor activities when the pollen count is high.
- If freshly cut grass triggers your symptoms, ask another family member to cut the grass, or hire an enterprising neighborhood youngster.
- Eliminate compost heaps or any piles of rotting leaves, ripe locations for the development of mold spores.
- Check the air-quality forecast if you live in an urban area where pollution is a problem. If the pollution index is high, spend as much of your day as possible inside with the air-conditioning on.
- Do not use pesticides to treat your lawn or garden. Because these chemicals can be potent triggers of asthma, look into natural alternatives, such as planting flowers that naturally repel insects.
- If cold air is a trigger for your asthma, you have two options. On some occasions you may choose to stay inside; at other times, when you know you will be exposed to cold air, your doctor may recommend that you use medication prior to exposure to prevent symptoms.
- Wear a mask or cover your nose and mouth with a scarf to keep cold air from triggering your asthma.

If You Have a Pet

If your asthma is triggered by animal dander or feathers, your best bet is to find another home for the household cat, dog, hamster, or bird that is causing symptoms. Asthma may become a problem even when exposure to common allergens such as dust mites is low, when children are exposed and sensitized to cats and dogs at an early age.

Many people with asthma are emotionally attached to their pets. Asthmatics who choose not to part with cherished household pets can take other measures to limit their exposure to pet allergens:

- Keep the pet outdoors as much as possible.
- Wash and brush the pet frequently.
- Ban the pet from the bedroom.
- Avoid using flea collars or powders that are packed with dangerous chemicals. When you pet your cat or dog, these chemicals can get on your hands and cause asthma symptoms. Natural flea controls, available at most local pet stores, are a safer alternative for both you and the animal you care for.

When You Travel

If you have asthma, there are two small words that best arm you for travel: be prepared. If you're susceptible to pollen, determine what the pollen count will be at your destination. If cold air is a trigger, check the weather. Have backup medications and instructions on how to use them close at hand. The following tips can help you prepare for travel, so that you can relax and enjoy your trip:

- At all times, keep in mind what triggers your asthma, and take precautions to avoid triggers when you travel.

- Be sure to pack a sufficient supply of medication and keep it readily accessible. Metered-dose inhalers are as convenient to tuck in your bag as a bottle of pills or capsules.
- Carry your peak-flow meter, and remember to monitor regularly how well you're breathing.
- If you have severe asthma, you may want to consider traveling with a nebulizer, an electronic device that can rapidly deliver medications such as cromolyn and beta-agonists into the lungs. It may also be wise to carry prednisone with you.
- Wear a Medic Alert bracelet in case of emergency. Ask your doctor to write out specific instructions for emergency treatment.
- Take a close look at your destination. For instance, if you're sensitive to air pollutants, a destination such as Los Angeles is not the best choice for your summer vacation.

Hotels, Motels, and Inns

- Make sure you're registered on a no-smoking floor.
- Book reservations in establishments that are clean and free of asthma-inducing dust and molds.
- Ask to see your room before you pay for it. If there is dust, mildew, or cigarette smoke, switch to another room or a different hotel.

On the Road

- If you travel during pollen season, keep the car windows closed and the air conditioner on.
- Also in pollen season, set your air conditioner to recirculate air in the car. Do not open the vent, which will allow pollen to enter the car.
- If your asthma is severe or unpredictable, consider investing in a portable nebulizer, which can be charged with the cigarette lighter in your car.
- Don't use moldy, dirty bathrooms in service stations. Take advantage of clean rest stops.
- Don't allow anyone to smoke in your car.

Air Travel

- When you fly, your medication should be in your carry-on bag—not in the baggage compartment, where it can do you no good if symptoms occur.
- Airlines sometimes cut back on air-conditioning when the plane is waiting to take off or land. If this happens on your plane, inform the flight attendant that you have asthma and may develop symptoms under these conditions. You can hope that the air-conditioning will come back on—if it doesn't, be prepared to use your metered-dose inhaler.
- Call the airline a day ahead and order a special fruit or vegetarian meal. Regular airline food is often processed and may be packed with tartrazine or sulfites.

International Travel

- Although smoking is banned on domestic flights, it is still permitted on many international flights. Be certain you are seated in the no-smoking section, far removed from the smoking area.
- Be especially careful when ordering meals in other countries. You will probably be unaware of all the ingredients in the food you eat, some of which may be potential triggers. Order simple, recognizable foods.
- If you use a nebulizer, be sure to pack a converter.

Asthma Camps for Children

Traveling can pose special obstacles for children. Registering asthmatic children in a summer asthma camp can help them both physically and psychologically, while the medical supervision at asthma camps can give parents peace of mind.

Summers at asthma camp, in the company of other asthmatic children, are often recommended by doctors to help children hone their coping skills, receive emotional support from others who share their condition, and engage in all kinds of outdoor activities in a secure, medically supervised environment.

Asthma summer camps can build self-reliance, self-esteem, and physical self-assurance in your child. (For more information about summer camps for children, turn to Chapter 5. Call your American Lung Association chapter for information about asthma summer camps in your area.)

CHAPTER 8

Using Medications

Asthma treatment has advanced dramatically over the past few years. Only a decade ago, the care of asthma focused primarily on treating bronchospasm. Bronchodilators were used to relieve the breathlessness, wheezing, coughing, and chest tightness of acute attacks. Asthmatics who carried a bronchodilator in their pockets were led mistakenly to believe that their asthma was under control.

More recently, scientists have discovered that the underlying cause or condition of asthma—the inflammation and swelling of the linings of twitchy airways—may actually be the most common feature, and potentially greatest danger, of asthma. Inflammation often leads to the development of asthmatic symptoms and, when left uncontrolled, may cause permanent lung damage. The good news is that using anti-inflammatory drugs regularly, even when symptoms are not present, can reduce inflammation and hyperreactivity in the airways.

Today there are a variety of safe and effective medications to help asthmatics control both the symptoms themselves and the conditions in the airways that allow those symptoms to occur. There is no one best medication routine for asthmatics: doctors tailor treatment to fit each individual's needs, often combining different drugs to get the best results. Depending on the frequency and severity of your symptoms, your physician will recommend that you take asthma medications routinely or as needed.

Whatever medication you take for your asthma, there are some basic guidelines that will help you medicate safely and wisely. Pay close attention to the prescription amounts and schedules set by your physician, and take care not to skip doses. Remember to ask about potential problems, such as drug interactions and side effects, and be certain to inform your doctor immediately if you experience an adverse reaction. Your physician should take the time to explain these things to you, and to be available to answer your questions. (For more tips on how to take medication, see "Taking Responsibility" at the end of this chapter.)

The Two Types of Asthma Medications

Anti-inflammatory and bronchodilator drugs are the two types of medications most commonly chosen to treat asthma today. Anti-inflammatories are taken to prevent the symptoms of asthma; bronchodilators are used to manage symptoms when they occur. When exercise is a trigger, bronchodilators can prevent symptoms if taken approximately fifteen minutes before you begin your workout.

There are two leading types of asthma medications:

• Anti-inflammatory drugs stabilize the basophils, or mast cells, which release inflammatory chemicals when exposed to triggers. A lesser degree of inflammation in the airways means fewer asthmatic episodes and a reduced possibility of permanent lung damage caused by chronic or uncontrolled inflammation. Anti-inflammatories should be taken regularly, according to your doctor's instructions, whether or not symptoms are present.

• Bronchodilators quickly open blocked airways. Doctors use these medications to manage acute asthma attacks, as well as to relax the small, smooth muscles that tighten around airways and block the flow of air in and out of the lungs.

Anti-Inflammatory Medications

The use of anti-inflammatory drugs as a preventive measure is the cornerstone of asthma therapy today. Because they are preventive, don't skip doses of medication—no matter how well you feel. Routine use of anti-inflammatory drugs can help prevent the inflammation that may lead to chronic symptoms or asthma attacks.

Following are descriptions of the most common anti-inflammatory medications used in the treatment of asthma.

Corticosteroids

Corticosteroids, also known simply as steroids, are the most effective anti-inflammatory drugs for the care of asthma. They are available in three forms: inhaled, oral, and by injection. Regular use of inhaled corticosteroids is by far the safest method, while short bursts of oral steroids are also extremely effective. Injectable steroids are less common as a regular treatment.

The adrenal glands in your body naturally produce many different hormones called steroids. Corticosteroids, the type of steroids used to treat asthma, are chemical derivatives of a human hormone produced by your body's adrenal gland. These are NOT the same steroids that are banned for use by Olympic athletes; the steroids taken by athletes are anabolic steroids, which increase muscle mass but may harm the liver and impair fertility.

Corticosteroids act to reduce and prevent inflammation in the airways of your lungs. They also decrease hyperreactivity of airways, and can relieve wheezing. Until recent years, only oral corticosteroids were available, and these were usually reserved for the treatment of very severe cases of asthma. Members of the cortisone family, these drugs have very serious side effects, especially when taken over long periods. Because of this, physicians in the past were reluctant to prescribe them.

Today corticosteroids are available in inhaled as well as oral and injected forms. Inhaled corticosteroids can be taken directly into the lungs, thus avoiding the dangerous side effects that may occur if they enter the bloodstream. Oral corticosteroids continue to be prescribed in short bursts to control serious cases of asthma—but with the caution that is demanded of a medication with such serious side effects.

Inhaled Corticosteroids

Inhaled corticosteroids safely and effectively prevent inflammation and decrease hyperreactivity in the bronchial tubes. When they are used properly, there is an increased absorption of medication into the lung tissue, while medication is prevented from entering the bloodstream. This significantly reduces the risk of the adverse side effects usually associated with corticosteroids.

Inhaled corticosteroids include triamcinolone (Azmacort), flunisolide (AeroBid), and beclomethasone (Vanceril and Beclovent). A built-in spacing device makes Azmacort especially convenient to use. (Read about the proper use of metered-dose inhalers and spacing devices later in this chapter.)

Rinsing your mouth after using inhaled medications is an easy way to prevent most side effects. Possible side effects of inhaled corticosteroids include:

- Occasional coughing
- Hoarseness
- Thrush, or a yeast infection in the mouth

Oral Corticosteroids

Oral corticosteroids, such as prednisone (Deltasone) and methylprednisolone (Medrol), are an especially effective treatment for severe cases of asthma. Tablets begin to take effect some three hours after you take them, lessening airway inflammation and excessive mucus production, and allowing bronchodilators to work more efficiently. The use of five- to eight-day bursts of oral steroids is appropriate, and can prevent asthmatic patients from having to visit the doctor's office or emergency room.

Oral corticosteroids can lead to major side effects, which is why these drugs are prescribed with extreme caution. Even short-term use of oral corticosteroids may result in adverse reactions, such as bloating and weight gain. Long-term use increases the risk of serious health problems, including osteoporosis, hypertension, and cataracts.

Because of these potential problems, oral corticosteroids are usually prescribed in short-term bursts of several days to several weeks. When they are used for these limited periods, side effects such as fluid retention and increased appetite are temporary and disappear when the medication is stopped. Only in very severe cases of asthma—when the risk of dangerous side effects is outweighed by the drug's prevention of life-threatening symptoms—are oral corticosteroids recommended as part of routine treatment. Whenever possible, oral corticosteroid therapy should be reduced by therapy with inhaled corticosteroids or other medications.

The use of oral corticosteroids has been associated with many adverse side effects, such as:

- Weight gain
- Fluid retention
- Bloating and rounding of the face
- Thinning of the skin
- Stomach upset and peptic ulcer

- Reduced resistance to disease (weakened immune system)
- Muscle weakness
- Easy bruising
- Osteoporosis
- Hypertension
- Cataracts
- Stunted growth in children

Cromolyn Sodium

Cromolyn sodium, which is sold under the brand name Intal, is a safe and effective preventive treatment for asthma. Cromolyn controls symptoms triggered by allergies, cold air, and exercise. It appears to work by stabilizing and preventing the release of inflammatory mediators (such as histamine) from mast cells.

At least two or three weeks of therapy are usually necessary before cromolyn takes effect. Although cromolyn is generally considered safer than inhaled corticosteroids, it is also more expensive.

Cromolyn has been associated with few side effects, although users may occasionally experience coughing or a sore throat.

Nedocromil Sodium

Nedocromil sodium, which is sold under the brand name Tilade, is very similar to cromolyn. This is a new drug on the market, so fewer asthmatics may be familiar with it; some people who have tried it seem to object to its taste. Nedocromil prevents asthma symptoms by reducing underlying inflammation in the airways.

Like cromolyn, nedocromil has been associated with only minor side effects, especially coughing and sore throat.

Bronchodilators

Bronchodilators open up, or dilate, bronchioles. They relax the muscles around airways, allowing air to move more freely in and out of the lungs. Bronchodilators are usually taken in inhaled form, through metered-dose inhalers or nebulizers, to relieve the shortness of breath, tight chest, coughing, and wheezing of an asthma attack. Bronchodilator medication is also available in controlled-release or timed-action capsules and tablets for maintenance therapy in severe cases of asthma.

While bronchodilators provide fast and effective relief of severe symptoms, their role in asthma management programs is being reassessed. Many experts warn of "bronchodilator abuse," meaning overuse. Because bronchodilators relieve troubling symptoms, they enable asthmatics to tolerate exposure to allergens, irritants, and other triggers of asthma that can damage the lungs. Overuse of these drugs may lull you into a false sense of security. They may lead you to ignore the valuable natural warning signs (that is, your symptoms) that essentially tell you to get out of the way of potentially harmful substances.

Still, when properly used, bronchodilators continue to play a valuable role in asthma management. Even when triggers are avoided and preventive anti-inflammatory medication is taken, asthma symptoms may still occur.

Bronchodilators provide fast and effective relief of troubling symptoms, and are also helpful as a pre-exercise asthma deterrent.

Following are descriptions of the most common bronchodilator medications used in the treatment of asthma.

Beta-Agonists

Beta-agonists are considered the medications of choice for the treatment of asthma attacks. Inhaled beta-agonists take effect immediately, relaxing constriction in airways. Medications in this group include albuterol (Proventil, Ventolin), bitolterol (Tornalate), metaproterenol (Alupent, Metaprel), pirbuterol (Maxair), and terbutaline (Brethaire, Brethine, Bricanyl).

Salmeterol (Serevent) is a newly released beta-agonist that differs from the others in that it lasts for 12 hours and therefore should not be used more than twice in one day; other beta-antagonists are effective for only 4 to 6 hours. Salmeterol may be especially useful for the treatment of nocturnal asthma. With rare exception, Severent should be used only by patients who are already taking an anti-inflamatory medication on a regular basis.

Beta-agonists can also be used regularly to help control chronic airway narrowing, and can be taken to prevent episodes of exercise-induced asthma. The inhaled forms of beta-agonists are usually preferable to tablets, since they have the advantage of working immediately and causing fewer side effects.

Moderate use of beta-agonists, as directed by your doctor, is usually not associated with long-term side effects. Side effects of beta-agonist drugs can include:

- Tremor
- Dizziness

- Rapid heartbeat
- Anxiety and nervousness
- Elevated blood pressure

Theophylline

Theophylline is one of the most frequently used asthma medications. It acts by relaxing bronchial muscles, thus opening blocked airways and making it easier to breathe. Theophylline is sold under more than fifty brand names, including Aerolate, Constant-T, Respbid, Slo-bid, Slo-Phyllin, Sustaine, Theo-24, Theobid, Theochron, Theo-dur, Theolair, Theovent, and Uniphyl.

Recent concern has focused on safety questions about theophylline. Its potential for adverse side effects—coupled with the development of safer yet still effective medications—has meant that theophylline, while still an important drug in the treatment of asthma, is prescribed less frequently and more cautiously than in the past.

Theophylline is available in tablet, capsule, or liquid form. Most people prefer the tablets or capsules, since the liquid has a disagreeable taste. Sustained-release preparations of theophylline, such as Slo-bid and Theo-dur, are effective for longer periods than inhaled beta-agonists, which make them especially useful in the treatment of nocturnal, or nighttime, asthma. Your doctor may recommend that you take tablets or capsules at bedtime. (Theophylline liquid is not available in this long-acting form.) This way theophylline will reach peak effectiveness in the early-morning hours, when asthma symptoms are most likely to bother you.

An advantage of theophylline is that your physician

can monitor its level in your blood. The rate of absorption of this drug into the bloodstream varies from person to person. Children, for example, rapidly eliminate theophylline from their bodies; physical conditions such as congestive heart failure and interaction with certain drugs such as erythromycin, on the other hand, slow the elimination of theophylline, causing theophylline levels to rise. Appropriate dosages of theophylline, and careful monitoring of its level in your blood, are helpful in ensuring that this medication is acting effectively within its therapeutic range.

Theophylline is in the same family as caffeine and, like coffee and other caffeine products, is associated with central nervous system stimulation. Possible side effects of theophylline include:

- Nausea and vomiting
- Fast or irregular heartbeat
- Stomachache and diarrhea
- Headaches
- Restlessness and irritability
- Loss of appetite
- Insomnia
- Muscle twitching
- Seizures
- Behavioral disturbances in children

Anticholinergics

In the past, the anticholinergic agent atropine was a popular treatment for asthma. But when atropine proved slower to take effect and had more side effects than newer beta-agonist bronchodilators, emphasis shifted away from anticholinergics. The development of the new anticholinergic ipratropium (Atrovent), however, has renewed interest in this type of medication.

Inhaled anticholinergics act by blocking reflexes in the nerves which control bronchial muscles. By blocking these reflexes, which are usually triggered by inhaled irritants, anticholinergic drugs control the smooth-muscle contractions that bring on wheezing, breathlessness, and other symptoms of asthma.

Ipratropium (Atrovent) has few side effects. Occasional difficulties include a cough and dry mouth.

Inhalers and Nebulizers

Some asthma medications are taken orally, but drugs such as beta-agonists and cromolyn are inhaled into the lungs through metered-dose inhalers and nebulizers. Breathing in medication is an effective way of getting it directly to the airways where it is needed while avoiding entrance into the bloodstream, where it can lead to adverse side effects. The effectiveness of inhaled medication depends on the proper use of the metered-dose inhalers or nebulizers through which it is taken.

How to Use a Metered-Dose Inhaler

- Remove the inhaler cap and set the inhaler upright.
- Shake the inhaler.
- Tilt your head back and exhale.

- Place the inhaler an inch in front of your open mouth.
- Press down on the inhaler, releasing medication as you breathe in.
- Breathe in slowly and evenly for three to five seconds.
- Hold your breath for ten seconds, so that medication can settle on the airway linings.
- Repeat puffs as directed by your doctor.

Spacer Devices

Many people, especially children and the elderly, find metered-dose inhalers somewhat difficult to use. Attaching a spacer device can simplify the use of an MDI. A spacer provides a reservoir into which the appropriate amount of medication is released before use, thus eliminating the need to coordinate the inhalation just right. Spacers are also helpful when taking inhaled steroids, since it is especially important to get steroids directly into the airways to avoid adverse side effects.

How to Use a Nebulizer

Nebulizers, or air compressors, provide even easier delivery of inhaled medications. Medication is placed in a canister attached to a face mask or mouthpiece and is nebulized into a fine mist, which can be easily inhaled. Nebulizers are especially useful for getting medication into small children. They're also helpful in cases of severe asthma, where attacks occur frequently or unpredictably.

Nebulizers are widely available in emergency rooms for treatment of asthma attacks, and now they are available for home use as well. Parents of asthmatic children may want to invest in their own nebulizer, and people with severe asthma may find it useful to travel with portable nebulizers. Though more expensive than MDIs, nebulizers are covered by most health plans. Ask your doctor whether a nebulizer is appropriate for your asthma.

Inhaler Overuse

As we mentioned earlier, while inhaled bronchodilator medications are a boon in the treatment of asthma, inhaler overuse is inhaler abuse. If you use your MDI or nebulizer too frequently, you may only be delaying the treatment of dangerous underlying inflammation in your airways. Irregular heartbeat may also result from overuse of inhalers. Be sure you consult your physician about the amount of inhaler use that is right for you.

Emergency Medication

When normal treatment of asthma is not enough to relieve symptoms, an emergency trip to the doctor's office or hospital is necessary for more intensive asthma management. A situation in which the symptoms of your asthma become unusually severe and do not respond to routine measures—when your asthma is out of control and life-threatening—is known as status asthmaticus. Because this can be a very alarming and distressing experience, it's best to prepare for the possibility of its occurring. Knowing what to expect can subtract much of the potential fear and anxiety from the situation.

An injection of a fast-acting bronchodilator such as epinephrine (Adrenalin) or terbutaline (Brethine or Bricanyl) is a very common emergency treatment of status asthmaticus. These drugs immediately open blocked airways, providing relief of severe asthma symptoms within minutes. However, be sure to inform the emergency room doctor if you have high blood pressure, a thyroid condition, or heart problems; epinephrine has a strong effect on your heart, and under these circumstances should probably not be used. Headache and nausea are also common side effects of epinephrine. Fortunately, safer alternatives are available.

Today nebulizer treatments are being used more and more frequently in emergencies. They provide quick relief of a sudden or unexpected asthma attack, without the potential side effects of injected bronchodilators. Using a nebulizer to inhale a bronchodilator—such as a metaproterenol (Alupent or Metaprel) or albuterol (Proventil or Ventolin)—has less effect on the heart and does not cause the shakiness associated with injected epinephrine.

Emergency treatment of status asthmaticus may also include oxygen therapy, through either a mask or a nasal tube. Doctors may follow up initial treatment with intravenous solutions of theophylline or corticosteroids. Tests may be taken, such as a chest X ray to assess possible complications of asthma. Throughout emergency treatment, the doctor will use spirometry, or breathing tests, to measure the extent of airway blockage.

You will need to take extra medications for some time after an asthma attack, until your lungs gradually return to normal. The best way to avoid a repeat of status asthmaticus is to learn to recognize the warning signs of asthma attacks, and take early measures to avoid them or lessen their severity. (Refer to Chapter 4 for a detailed list of the warning signs of an asthma attack.)

Taking Responsibility

Once your doctor has given you a prescription, it is up to you to follow through with taking medication correctly. Some basic guidelines can help you medicate safely and wisely. Follow your doctor's directions exactly; never change your medication program without discussing it with your doctor. Always inform your doctor if you are breast-feeding, pregnant, or thinking about becoming pregnant; drugs can negatively affect a growing baby or developing fetus.

Do not skip preventive doses of medication, and be certain you know what medication to take if you experience an asthma attack. Remember that the worst thing you can do during an attack is panic. Shortness of breath, coughing, and wheezing can all worsen when you become anxious and upset. Once you understand what to do in case of emergency—to recognize the warning signs of an asthma episode and to take the appropriate medication prescribed by your physician—there is no need to get overanxious. Calm and efficient self-care is an important part of successful asthma management.

Don't hesitate to ask questions of your doctor, especially when starting a new medication. A good cooperative working relationship with your doctor is essential to effective management of asthma. It often helps to have your doctor put your medication regimen in writing; both you and those close to you will benefit from easy access to this information. In many cases, your pharmacist can also help out. Many pharmacies today keep computer records of the various medications their customers take, and pharmacists can inform you of possible interactions.

Following are some important questions to ask your doctor or pharmacist before taking any medication:

- What are the generic and brand names of the medication I am taking?
- What is the reason for taking this medication?
- How long must I use it before my symptoms are relieved?
- What should I do if the medication does not relieve my symptoms?
- Should I continue to take this medication even when I am no longer experiencing symptoms?
- How often should I take this medication?
- What is the proper dosage?
- Should I take this medication with meals or on an empty stomach?
- What should I do if I accidentally skip a dose?
- Will this medication interact with other prescription or over-the-counter medications I take?
- What side effects should I expect?
- What should I do if I experience an allergic or adverse reaction?

CHAPTER 9

The Importance of Exercise

Exercise is vital to our physical and psychological health, whether or not we have asthma. Yet for many years asthmatics were discouraged from engaging in vigorous exercise. A common myth was that asthmatics were "delicate" individuals, who could not excel or sometimes even participate in exercise and sports. This left many asthmatics—especially growing children who had asthma—at increased risk of becoming overweight and out of shape.

Today we have a far greater understanding of the relationship between asthma and exercise. It's increasingly apparent not only that people with asthma CAN exercise, but that if you have asthma, you *should* exercise. Asthma places extra physical and emotional demands on your body, and you must be in the best possible physical shape to cope with them. The fact that exercise can be a trigger of asthma symptoms is *not* a reason to forgo exercise; in the vast majority of cases, appropriate med-

ication can control exercise-induced asthma. Having
asthma hasn't prevented Olympic athletes—including
Jackie Joyner-Kersee, Jeanette Bolden, Nancy Hogs-
head, and Jim Ryun—from competing.

Exercise Your Way to Health

Exercise increases lung and heart fitness in people of
all ages. Regular exercise can help lower your blood
pressure and reduce atherosclerosis, which can lead to
heart disease. In fact, exercise carries an enormous
range of benefits to your whole body: when you work
out regularly, you'll find that you feel less fatigue, have
more energy, and enjoy more overall fitness. Exercise
can reduce your risk of heart attack, stroke, arthritis,
emphysema, and osteoporosis.

Exercise is also one of the best things you can do for
your asthma. Lung fitness is a clear priority when you
have asthma, and when you exercise regularly, exercise
may even boost your respiratory capacity.

Besides adding to your good physical health, exercise
contributes to your overall sense of well-being. It's one
of the best natural stress-busters available. It enables
you to relax and get a good night's sleep, and just
makes you feel better. It stimulates the release from
your brain of "feel good" endorphins, which can help
banish negative feelings such as fear or anxiety—
feelings you may sometimes experience when you have
asthma. Exercising as a member of a team can also help
build self-esteem.

Besides all these benefits, exercise helps you main-
tain strength and good posture. Strength may be an
issue for asthmatics who regularly take oral cortico-

steroids, which can interfere with their absorption of calcium and lead to brittle bones.

Getting Started

If you don't exercise regularly—that is, if you lead what's called a sedentary life—it's best to consult your doctor before embarking on an exercise program. After giving you a complete physical examination, your physician will no doubt recommend that you start gradually.

Swimming, walking, and stationary cycling are good exercises to begin with. Remember that it's important for everyone to begin an exercise program slowly and sensibly—especially for asthmatics, who are at risk of triggering sudden symptoms. So start small, and bit by bit you will build strength and endurance.

Exercise Can Trigger Asthma Symptoms

Exercise often leads to wheezing and coughing in people who have asthma. If exercise is a trigger of your asthma, your exercise program should be closely monitored by your doctor.

Because you breathe more rapidly through your mouth when you engage in continuous or particularly strenuous exercise, the air that reaches the bronchial tubes inside your lungs is not warmed and humidified as effectively as the air that normally enters through your nose. This cooler and drier air—often in combination with the larger amounts of air you take in while exercising—irritates the twitchy airways of many asthmatics and triggers symptoms.

Exercising in Cold Air

Exercising in cold weather can make matters even worse. If you have asthma, play it safe and check with your doctor before exercising in cold air. Exercise and cold air are both possible triggers of asthma attacks. In fact, the only time some asthmatics experience difficulty in breathing is when exercising during cold weather.

Wear a mask, muffler, or scarf over your face when you venture forth on a chilly winter day. Whether you are sledding, snowshoeing, or taking a peaceful walk in the woods, covering your face will help warm cold air before it reaches your sensitive bronchial tubes. Layering your clothes is a good idea for overall comfort.

If it's an especially cold and windy day, turn on the radio or TV and check the local weather before going out. When it's extremely cold outside—or when the wind-chill factor just makes it feel that way—you may want to take a day off from exercise, or choose to exercise indoors.

When natural preventive measures fail to help, your doctor will prescribe medication for exercise-induced asthma. Treatment with drugs can help virtually all asthmatics enjoy the exercise of their choice.

Preventing Exercise-Induced Asthma

Exercise is necessary and beneficial—especially if you have a chronic disease such as asthma—but should not be taken too casually. Exercise is a very common trigger of bronchospasm and other symptoms in people who have asthma.

For some people, exercise is the sole trigger of

asthma symptoms, while for others it is one of several triggers. Whatever triggers your asthma, virtually everyone with asthma should be able to participate in the activity of his or her choice.

If exercise is a trigger for your asthma, you can work with your doctor to learn how to pace yourself. Warming up before exercise—and cooling down afterward— can help ward off the symptoms of asthma. You can also take precautions to avoid irritations that may trigger an asthma attack. In most cases, this simply means using common sense. For example, don't go running on a hot and smoggy afternoon, or when the pollen count is high.

Medications for Exercise-Induced Asthma

In many cases, preventive measures alone are not enough to control exercise-induced asthma. Fortunately, medications are available to prevent and treat exercise-related asthma symptoms. Your doctor may prescribe medication for you to take before exercise to prevent symptoms, as well as backup bronchodilators to treat any symptoms you do experience. Discuss with your doctor which medications are right for you. Remember that asthma therapy should allow you to tolerate just about any form of exercise you like.

Following are the medications most frequently prescribed for exercise-related asthma.

Beta-Agonists

Beta-agonists are used regularly to prevent episodes of exercise-induced asthma. They work by preventing the narrowing of bronchial tubes that exercise triggers. Beta-agonists, such as albuterol and metaproterenol, can also be used to reverse bronchospasm that has been triggered by exercise.

Cromolyn Sodium

Cromolyn sodium is a very useful medication for the relief of asthma symptoms triggered by exercise and cold air. It works by stabilizing mast cells, preventing them from releasing mediators such as histamine. Although cromolyn's effect as an anti-inflammatory agent may take two or three weeks, it can be taken before exercise, as needed, and still be effective. However, it must be taken *before* exercise—it is not effective once asthma symptoms begin.

Theophylline

Theophylline acts by relaxing bronchial muscles, thus opening blocked airways and making it easier to breathe. When used as a regular daily medication, theophylline is often very effective in preventing exercise-induced asthma. It is not as effective as either inhaled beta-agonists or cromolyn when used as needed, because of its frequent side effects and slower action.

For more information on the medications used to treat asthma, turn to Chapter 8.

When to Consult an Asthma Specialist

Often people find that their primary-care physicians simply cannot control exercise-induced asthma. If this is the case with you, don't despair: consult an asthma specialist. In almost every case, a specialist can provide an aggressive medication program that will prevent or relieve your symptoms. And with aggressive management of your asthma, you can enjoy almost any exercise you wish.

Types of Exercise

As we've said again and again, aggressive management of your asthma should permit you to participate in virtually any exercise. Often swimming is cited as the ideal exercise for asthmatics, as the warm and humid conditions in which most swimming takes place are good for your airways. Exercise that occurs in short bursts, rather than sustained exercise, is also recommended by many doctors. But when your asthma is well managed, you should be able to engage in any exercise. While some doctors discourage activities such as running, keep in mind that runners who have asthma successfully compete in the Olympics.

There are many reasons we exercise: for endurance, for strength, for flexibility, for speed. All exercises are important for your overall health and peace of mind. Two categories of exercise that you as an asthmatic should include in your program are aerobic exercise and weight-bearing exercise.

Aerobic Exercise

Aerobic exercise, of prime importance to asthmatics, is excellent for all-around health and prevention. It builds your endurance, gets your heart and lungs pumping, improves your blood circulation, and sends oxygen to all the muscles in your body.

Aerobic exercise can help your asthma by improving your aerobic conditioning. Try to exercise at least four times a week for about forty minutes. If you're out of shape, start out with ten minutes three times a week and gradually lengthen your aerobic sessions. Warm up first to loosen your muscles, tendons, and ligaments; cool down after aerobic exercise to protect your muscles, reducing muscle tightness and the chance of cramps or spasms.

Aerobic activities include swimming, walking, jogging or running, dancing, rowing, cross-country skiing, and skating. Regular aerobic exercise can:

- Boost your respiratory capacity.
- Enhance cardiac function.
- Lower your total cholesterol.
- Improve your blood sugar level.
- Reduce high blood pressure.
- Eliminate excess body fat.
- Reduce your risk of stroke and heart attack.
- Clear your mind, relax you, and increase your self-esteem.

Weight-Bearing Exercise

Many people still continue to equate weight-bearing exercise—that is, exercising for strength—with acquiring the physique of a muscular bodybuilder. But strong muscles look better and work better in all of us. As with any new workout, however, be sure to consult your doctor before embarking on an exercise program of this type, and also advise your exercise instructor or coach if you are taking oral steroids.

There are three ways in which you can exercise for strength:

- Calisthenics, such as push-ups, sit-ups, leg raises, and body twists.
- Free weights, such as lifting dumbbells or barbells.
- Weight-bearing machines, such as the Nautilus and Universal systems you find in most health clubs and gyms today.

The philosophy of weight-bearing exercise is simple: reduce resistance and increase repetitions. In the Nautilus circuit training popular in many clubs today, you may lift a ten-pound weight twelve to fifteen times—not a thirty-pound weight twice. This technique builds muscles while minimizing stress on your circulation. As well as consulting your asthma doctor, be sure that you know the proper way to perform all exercises and use any equipment.

Weight-bearing exercises are particularly important for the small percentage of asthmatics who take oral corticosteroids regularly, since this type of medication regimen can interfere with the absorption of calcium.

Calcium is an essential mineral for strong teeth and bones, and is an important factor in blood, muscle, and nervous system functions. A lack of calcium can lead to brittle bones and osteoporosis; doing weight-bearing exercises regularly can help reverse this process.

Weight-bearing exercise is also increasingly important for women as they age. Women begin to lose bone mass around age thirty-five, and weight-bearing exercise builds bone and increases bone density. Doing weight-bearing exercises regularly can help prevent crippling osteoporosis in later years.

Exercise Safely

We hope you've learned one very important fact from this chapter: With effective management of your asthma, you should be able to participate in the exercise of your choice. Remember that it's also important to exercise safely and responsibly.

- Before beginning any exercise program, see your doctor and get a thorough physical examination.
- Set aside a regular time for exercise each day.
- Start slowly. If you've led a sedentary life, don't push yourself to accomplish too much too soon. You may end up jeopardizing your health rather than improving it.
- Make exercise part of your daily life. Take the stairs instead of the elevator, mow the lawn, or try walking part of the way to work.
- Set attainable goals. If you're like most people, you'll find that you're more likely to follow through on a realistic exercise program.

- Keep a journal of your exercise program to record your goals and your progress in meeting them. If you start out walking for ten minutes three times a week, you'll be amazed to discover how your endurance has increased and how many miles you've covered after a month.

- Be flexible. If you miss a day, it's not the end of the world. If you're ill or busy, cut back—don't try to pack your weekly exercise quota into one or two sessions. But do be sure to get back on track again as soon as you reasonably can.

- Exercise with a friend. Companionship can make exercise more enjoyable and help motivate you to follow through on your exercise resolutions.

- Choose exercises that are right for you. These are the exercises you enjoy most, and also the ones that fit most conveniently into your schedule.

- Always allow time to warm up and cool down. Warm-ups and cool-downs are a must if exercise is a trigger of your asthma.

- Exercise in appropriate weather. Heat, humidity, and air pollution can bring on asthma symptoms—as can cold, dry weather. On inclement days, either skip exercise or do it inside.

- If seasonal symptoms are a problem for you, be aware that you may need extra medication, or avoid exercising when the pollen count is high.

- Likewise, check the smog index when you exercise outside in a city.

- Dress appropriately. For asthmatics, this means covering your face with a scarf or muffler on chilly days.

- Make sure the exercise equipment you use is safe and reliable. When you are doing weight-bearing exercises, your sneakers should be well made and fit well. Whether you're running or biking, throw away worn-out shoes. Always wear a helmet when you bicycle.

- Once you've established a regular exercise routine, try to aim for a little variety. As well as being more apt to hold your interest, a variety of exercises will help you work different muscle groups and organs. A balanced fitness program can also help you achieve different health goals—such as increasing endurance, strength, and flexibility.

- Adjust your diet to your exercise program. Decrease your fat intake, and eat plenty of fresh fruits and vegetables and whole grains. It's also important to drink plenty of liquids when you exercise. (For more information on diet, see Chapter 10.)

The Role of Diet

Most individuals who have asthma have no problems with food. Contrary to what many people think, food is not nearly as common a trigger of asthma as airborne irritants (pollen, mold spores, house-dust mites, etc.) and upper-respiratory infections. Still, certain foods—and, even more so, the many chemicals that are added to food—can leave you wheezing, sneezing, or coughing. And for a very few asthmatics, food can lead to serious asthma attacks.

If you can identify the specific food, additive, or preservative that triggers your asthma symptoms, the best treatment is simply to avoid it. People who have identified a food sensitivity can then be educated consumers, making a special effort to read labels in the supermarket and ask questions at restaurants.

Asthmatics generally have the same nutritional needs and food considerations as anyone else, but if you have asthma it's important to make a nutritious diet part of your day-to-day life. When it is not well controlled, asthma can place additional stress on your body. This is especially true for the small percentage of asthmatics who require regular treatment with oral corticosteroids, which can deplete the body of important nutrients. In general, remember that a variety of whole foods packed with vitamins and minerals is vital to everyone's good health.

Food and Asthmatic Reactions

Asthmatic reactions to food can vary widely. When a problem food is eaten, you may experience symptoms such as coughing, wheezing, shortness of breath, and tightness in the chest. Scientists caution that asthmatics are usually allergic to only one food, or at most two or three foods. It's a common misconception that people are sensitive or allergic to a wide variety of foods.

Both whole and processed foods can cause asthmatic reactions. If you're sensitive to shrimp, for example, be careful to avoid the many appetizers (egg rolls, stuffed mushrooms, etc.) that are likely to contain this shellfish. If chemical additives in food bother you, don't eat processed foods that contain them. Again, the best treatment is avoidance. The better the job you do in avoiding the triggers of your asthma, the easier it will be to control your condition.

Foods themselves, the chemicals that have been added to them, and individual susceptibility all play a role in determining whether or not you will experience an asthmatic reaction to a certain food. Even the time of year may play a part; when you're suffering a seasonal allergy such as hay fever, you may be extra sensitive to foods that are not ordinarily a problem for you.

Food seems to cause more asthmatic reactions in the very young. In many cases, this is a result of an infant's or toddler's inability to completely digest food proteins. Their small bodies perceive these partially digested food proteins as invaders and manufacture IgE antibodies to fight them. This causes allergic reactions in children, and one possible allergic reaction is asthma. Fortunately, many infants and toddlers who are sensitive or allergic to food products will be able to tolerate these foods as they grow older.

Allergy or Sensitivity?

The food allergy/sensitivity question is a great source of controversy in the study and treatment of food-related asthma. Current research indicates that many asthmatic reactions to food are the result of food *sensitivity*, or intolerance, rather than a true IgE-related or allergic response.

In any case, food sensitivity is so similar to food allergy that it is often difficult to make the distinction. In both instances histamine is released, which causes asthmatic reaction: symptoms such as difficulty in breathing, wheezing, coughing, tightened chest, and mucus production. The bottom line is that whether your reactions are due to food sensitivity or food allergy, the best thing that you can do is *identify* and *avoid* the foods that disturb you.

Chemicals in Food

If you have asthma, you may be neither sensitive nor allergic to any particular food—yet chemicals in the food you eat may irritate your sensitive airways. Food today is grown with the use of agricultural chemicals, and chemical additives and preservatives are added to many foods on grocery-store shelves. Chemicals in food and beverages can be a trigger of asthma symptoms:

- About 10 percent of asthmatics are sensitive to aspirin—and if you are sensitive to aspirin, you may be sensitive as well to tartrazine (Yellow Food Dye No. 5). Tartrazine is sometimes found in baked goods, cake mixes, candy, potato chips, pudding, soft drinks, and many other processed foods. Tartrazine and other food dyes may also be in medications such as antibiotics and birth control pills.

- In response to the health concerns of consumers, sulfites can no longer be applied to fruits and vegetables to keep them looking fresh. It's safe to go back to the salad bar. Yet sulfites, another possible trigger of asthma, are still used to preserve food. Metabisulfite (sodium bisulfite), an especially common food preservative and asthma trigger, may still turn up in a variety of processed foods. If you are sensitive to sulfites, be sure to read labels and avoid foods that contain them.

Common Food Sensitivities

People can be sensitive to all kinds of foods, but certain things we eat and drink seem to cause asthmatic reactions more frequently than others. As you know by now, sensitivity can be a reaction to the foods themselves or to the chemicals that have been added to them.

There are any number of problem foods associated with asthma, including shrimp, peanuts and peanut butter, other nuts, milk, many cheeses, yogurt, eggs, fish, citrus fruits, soy, and wheat. Processed foods are often packed with potentially asthma-inducing additives.

If you believe that a food or foods is at the bottom of your asthma symptoms, it's important to see a board-certified allergist who can identify your food sensitivities. You can then develop a strategy to eliminate from your diet the food or foods to which you are sensitive.

Identifying Problem Foods

To determine the significance of a food problem, your allergist will first take a very detailed medical history and conduct a physical examination. Allergists can often pinpoint problem foods simply by detecting patterns in these records. Your allergist may also ask you to create a food dairy after symptoms occur. Occasionally, your allergist may put you on a restricted diet.

After taking a comprehensive medical history, the allergist may recommend selective skin or blood testing to document the presence of IgE antibodies to foods. The history will determine which diagnostic tools are necessary to confirm which foods cause symptoms. Following are techniques your allergist may use to determine food sensitivity:

- **Skin tests.** Scratch or prick skin tests, which are frequently used to detect inhaled allergens, can also document the presence of IgE antibodies to foods.
- **RAST test.** The RAST test (Radioallergosorbent Test) directly measures specific IgE antibodies in the blood.
- **Elimination Diets.** Your allergist may recommend that you eliminate from your diet foods that appear to cause symptoms. On the basis of an elimination diet, an allergist can often discover problem foods.
- **Challenge tests.** A challenge test involves reintroducing a food removed in your elimination diet in order to confirm that the suspected food is indeed the one responsible for causing your symptoms. A challenge should *not* be attempted if your food sensitivity brings on severe or life-threatening symptoms.

Controlling Food-Related Asthma

Avoidance is the safest and most effective way to control asthma symptoms triggered by food. Once you have identified the foods that trigger your asthmatic reactions, the next step is to devise strategies to eliminate them from your diet:

- Check the labels of food products to make sure they do not contain the food or food additive to

which you are sensitive. If you are sensitive to
milk, for example, you should also avoid eating ice
cream, cheese, and milk chocolate, all of which
contain milk.

- When in doubt about ingredients, ask your grocer
  to explain them.
- If you are sensitive to food additives, don't be
  afraid to ask whether they have been used in the
  preparation of dishes you order in restaurants.
- Ask your pharmacist whether the medications you
  take include additives to which you are sensitive.
  If they do, consult your physician about prescrib-
  ing or recommending an alternative medication.
- If agricultural chemicals are found to be a trigger
  for your asthma, shop at natural-food stores and
  include more organic produce in your diet.

Asthma Medications and Your Diet

Although most asthma medications are safe and effective, it's important to be aware that the long-term use
of oral corticosteroids can lead to a calcium deficiency.
Such deficiency increases your risk of osteoporosis, a
crippling disease of brittle bones to which women are
especially susceptible. Calcium is essential for building
and maintaining strong bones and teeth.

Healthful and natural sources of calcium are low-fat
milk, yogurt, and cheese; and green vegetables such as
broccoli and spinach. Canned salmon and sardines,
which include crushed bones, are also rich sources of
calcium. In some cases, your doctor may recommend a
calcium supplement.

Nutritional Supplements

Asthmatics have the same basic nutritional requirements as other people. Still, when you have a chronic disease like asthma, your body may be under some additional stress. Sometimes, as we mentioned above, medications sap your body of valuable vitamins and minerals. Because of this, in addition to a good, sound diet, some doctors recommend that asthmatic patients take nutritional supplements. If you feel run-down—if you are ill, or traveling, or for some other reason are unable to meet your nutritional requirements—ask your physician whether a nutritional supplement is right for you.

CHAPTER 11

In the Future

We've come a long way from the time when asthma was considered a psychosomatic disease suffered by the high-strung children of overprotective mothers. Exciting new developments in research and clinical treatment of asthma continue to emerge every day. Clues to the cause of asthma are accumulating through genetic research, while newer and safer medications become available.

Genes that Affect Asthma

A revolution in the understanding of genetics is upon us; advances in molecular genetics are transforming the theory and practice of medicine today. Progress is being made at a dizzying rate.

Asthma, as we know, is an inherited disease, and advances in the science of genetics have made it possible to find the genes that predispose people to many diseases. Researchers have yet to find the genes that predispose people to develop asthma, but many current studies focus on them.

Gene therapy is also being tested to correct the many inherited gene mutations that cause asthma and other diseases. State-of-the-art research techniques include molecular modeling, in which drugs are designed on a computer. In studies of gene-splicing, fabricated genes instruct simple organisms to produce needed proteins. Researchers hope some day to convert the results of these studies into practical, clinical applications of gene therapy to asthma and other illnesses.

Asthma Is a Chronic Disease

As you've seen in the preceding pages, doctors today believe that too much emphasis has been placed on the use of bronchodilators to relieve asthma attacks. In response to current research, the National Institutes of Health has redefined asthma as a chronic rather than an acute disease.

While bronchodilators continue to play an invaluable role in easing the symptoms of asthma, the hallmark of asthma therapy today is using anti-inflammatory drugs to prevent those symptoms from occurring in the first place. By controlling the underlying inflammation and irritation of airways in the lungs, the vast majority of asthmatics can enjoy a full and active life.

Moving and Asthma

Once, people with asthma or allergies saved their dollars to migrate to Southwestern states in quest of cleaner air. When they retired, our parents did it for their health; parents of young asthmatic children today may consider making the same decision. But the truth is, it's not a good idea to move to a different part of the country simply because of your asthma or your allergies.

Today we realize that there is no ideal location for asthmatics. Initially a relocation may appear to cause an improvement in asthma symptoms, as the patient may have succeeded in evading triggers of asthma symptoms. But if you have the underlying twitchy airways that predispose you to developing asthma—or if you are prone to developing allergies, which can act as a trigger of asthma symptoms—moving is often not the answer. You may simply develop familiar symptoms in response to new stimuli. It's best to consult your physician and thoroughly research a new location before making a move.

Alternative Treatments of Asthma

The best approach to asthma—and the one we emphasize in this book—consists of aggressive medical treatment and educated self-management. Yet many people with asthma become frustrated if their symptoms are not properly managed, and are tempted to explore alternatives to regular medical care. The problem may actually be that you do not have the right doctor;

referral to an asthma specialist is often the solution to problems with asthma management and education.

As a well-informed consumer, you should be wary of alternative treatments that claim instant cures for asthma. Asthma is a chronic, usually lifelong condition that requires consistent, aggressive medical treatment and lifestyle management, such as avoiding triggers.

Nonetheless, some alternative strategies for dealing with asthma have merit. Because asthma is a serious condition, do not attempt any alternative strategies without first consulting your regular physician. In addition, alternative treatments should be viewed as a complement to rather than a replacement of conventional treatment. Following is a summary of the more common alternative approaches to asthma.

Acupuncture

Acupuncture is based on the theory that illness is the result of an imbalance in the energies that flow through your body. In this Chinese medical treatment, long, thin needles are inserted into specific points on the body to stabilize the flow of energy and relieve the symptoms of asthma and other diseases. Scientific evidence suggests that acupuncture may have some value in improving respiration.

Chiropractic

This medical practice presumes that the nervous system integrates all the body's functions. Chiropractors make "adjustments" to the body to improve asthma.

Some chiropractors appear to achieve success in treating asthma by reducing stress, which can trigger symptoms.

Herbalism

The use of herbs—remedies prepared from roots, leaves, and other parts of plants—is an age-old way in which you can both increase your overall resistance to disease and hasten your recovery from all types of illness. Ephedra, or ma huang, is the classic herbal remedy for asthma. Lobelia and elecampane are also beneficial lung tonics. Remedies such as these should be taken only under the supervision of an herbally oriented physician.

Holism

A holistic approach to health care addresses the physical, emotional, and spiritual aspects of healing. Health is viewed as a positive state, not merely as the absence of disease. Emphasis is placed on prevention and self-management. Holistic healers advise strategies such as relaxation practices and breathing exercises to aid asthmatics. Eliminating dairy products from the diet and taking B-complex vitamins are also common suggestions.

Homeopathy

Homeopathy is based on the idea that "like cures like." This is actually the same premise as immunotherapy, a series of allergy shots used to treat asthmatics for whom allergies are a trigger. (For more information on immunotherapy, turn to Chapter 8.) In homeopathy, symptoms are relieved by administering small, diluted solutions of the agent that produces the symptoms of the disease. The goal is gradual desensitization. Asthmatics should explore these types of remedies only under the care of an experienced homeopath.

The Self-Management of Asthma

The new medical understanding and treatments of asthma are extremely important. But if you have asthma, it's also imperative that you learn as much as you can about your own condition. This new trend in asthma is known as self-management or self-care.

You and your doctor can work as a team to identify the triggers of your asthma; then you can take an active role in eliminating your exposure to them. Even if you can't avoid every possible irritant outdoors and in, you can take valuable steps such as asthma-proofing your bedroom. You can aggressively monitor your own asthma by recognizing the warning signs of asthma and taking medications to prevent symptoms from occurring. In some cases, your doctor may recommend that you use a peak-flow meter to monitor your asthma.

The most important thing to realize is that you are a completely normal person who just happens to have asthma. When your asthma is managed appropriately, you can sleep through the night, get up and go to work or school, eat dinner, play ball, or work out—just like everybody else. Aggressive medical treatment and effective self-management can give you, the asthmatic, the tools with which to live a long, healthy, active, and normal life.

CHAPTER 12

For More Information

General Resources

Organizations

Allergy and Asthma Network/Mothers of
  Asthmatics
3554 Chain Bridge Road, Suite 200
Fairfax, VA 22030–2709
800–878–4403

Send a business-size, self-addressed envelope with fifty-two cents postage to receive a valuable information packet. Materials include the pamphlet "A Parent's Guide to Asthma" and referrals to asthma support groups for parents and summer camps especially for asthmatic children.

American Academy of Allergy and Immunology
611 East Well Street
Milwaukee, WI 53202
800–822–2762

Provides informative pamphlets as well as referrals to allergy specialists in your area.

American Academy of Allergy and Immunology
800 East Northwest Highway
Palatine, IL 60067
800–842–7777

Not affiliated with the organization of the same name listed above. Provides free information and referrals.

American College of Allergy and Immunology
85 West Algonquin Road, Suite 550
Arlington Heights, IL 60005
708–427–1200

This organization provides a number of helpful publications free of charge. General advice on asthma and allergies is available, as well as specific information on drugs used to treat asthma, exercise suggestions for asthmatics, and practical tips for pregnant patients.

American Lung Association
1740 Broadway
New York, NY 10019
212–315–8700

Provides free educational material about asthma and other lung diseases. Look in your local telephone directory for the address and phone number of the branch nearest you.

Asthma Allergy Foundation of America
1125 15th Street, N.W.
Washington, DC 20005
800–727–8462

Leave your name and address on their answering machine and they will send you a free information packet. Materials include a two-page instruction format for your asthmatic child's teacher that outlines your child's medication plan, what triggers asthma attacks in your child, and what to do in case of emergency.

National Asthma Education Program
   Information Center
4733 Bethesda Avenue
Bethesda, MD 20814
301–951–3260

Provides a number of free publications both for individuals and for school personnel.

National Jewish Center for Immunology
   and Respiratory Medicine
1400 Jackson Street
Denver, CO 80206
800–222–LUNG

One of the world's top medical centers for the treatment of asthma; it provides a number of free publications.

Recommended Reading

M. Eric Gershwin, M.D., and E. L. Klingelhofer, Ph.D., *Asthma: Stop Suffering, Start Living*. Reading, MA: Addison-Wesley, 1992.

National Institutes of Health, *Executive Summary: Guidelines for the Diagnosis and Management of Asthma*. Bethesda, MD: U.S. Department of Health and Human Services, 1991.

Thomas F. Plaut, M.D., *Children with Asthma: A Manual for Parents*. Amherst, MA: Pedipress, 1984.

Nancy Sander, *A Parent's Guide to Asthma: How You Can Help Your Child Control Asthma at Home, School, and Play*. New York: Plume, 1994.

Allan M. Weinstein, M.D., *Asthma: The Complete Guide to Self-Management of Asthma and Allergies for Patients and Their Families*. New York: Fawcett Crest, 1992.

Stuart H. Young, M.D., with Susan A. Shulman and Martin D. Shulman, Ph.D., *The Asthma Handbook*. New York: Bantam, 1989.

Suppliers of Products
for People with Asthma

Aller/Guard
1645 Southwest 41 Street
Topeka, KS 66609
800–234–0816

Allergy Clean Environments
125 Third Avenue
Haddon Heights, NJ 08035
800–882–4110

Allergy Control Products, Inc.
96 Danbury Road
P.O. Box 793
Ridgefield, CT 06877
800–422–DUST

Allergy Relief Shop
2932 Middlebrook Pike
Knoxville, TN 37921
800–678–2028

Allergy Research Group
P.O. Box 489
San Leandro, CA 94577
800–782–4274

The Allergy Store
P.O. Box 2555
Sebastopol, CA 95473
800–824–7163

AllerMed Corporation
31 Steel Road
Wylie, TX 75098
214–422–4898

Bio-Tech Systems
P.O. Box 25380
Chicago, IL 60625
800–621–5545

Mother Hart's Natural Products for Home and Body
P.O. Box 4229
Department PV
Boynton Beach, FL 33424
407–738–5866

National Allergy Supply
4400 Georgia Highway 120
Duluth, GA 30136
800–522–1448

SelfCare Catalog
5850 Shellmound Avenue
Emeryville, CA 94662
800–345–3371

Index

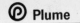

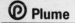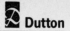